Cbd Oil

Naturally Heal Your Mental and Physical Health

(Your Natural Choice for Pain Relief and Living a Healthier and Happier Life)

Walter Koch

I0090261

Published By **Phil Dawson**

Walter Koch

All Rights Reserved

Cbd Oil: Naturally Heal Your Mental and Physical Health (Your Natural Choice for Pain Relief and Living a Healthier and Happier Life)

ISBN 978-1-7771462-3-8

Legal & Disclaimer

The information contained in this book is not designed to replace or take the place of any form of medicine or professional medical advice. The information in this book has been provided for educational & entertainment purposes only.

The information contained in this book has been compiled from sources deemed reliable, and it is accurate to the best of the Author's knowledge; however, the Author cannot guarantee its accuracy and validity and cannot be held liable for any errors or omissions. Changes are periodically made to this book. You must consult your doctor or get professional medical advice before using any of the suggested remedies, techniques, or information in this book.

Table Of Contents

Chapter 1: The Anatomy of Anxiety

We must begin with an idea of what anxiety is and the difference between it and anxiety. First step in taking control of any issue is to know what the issue is. A lot of times in day and age, we leap to the conclusion that it is and then implement the wrong solution to the problem, which only adds more stress to the already difficult problem.

CBD is a beneficial chemical for anxiety. But if aren't suffering from anxiety, or if you don't understand how to diagnose, or miss-interpret signs, you're in no position fix any issue. In this regard it is our intention to begin the chapter in this book exploring the nature and the nature of anxiety and in all forms.

The physiology of our body is always in some state or the other. If we're related to one another to each other, we're at a specific condition. If we feel scared that we're afraid, we're in a different place. If we're confused or troubled, then we're at a different level. A majority of states arises within us or through an external trigger. In that state, the way we perceive and view the world is influenced, shaped and coloured in that state.

Anxiety can be described as an emotional condition that manifests itself physically through physical manifestations and consequences. It's also a psychological condition that is triggered by traumatizing events. For example, soldiers have PTSD, which is a kind of anxiety.

Accordingly, anxiety could be described as a condition which affects the mental physical and emotional parts of an individual, causing the person to change their condition to become uncertain, chaotic, and ultimately destructive.

An underlying pattern of behaviour that includes apprehensive state of mind can develop into an habit that can cause symptoms that can disrupt everyday life for patients and others surrounding the patient. Ability to complete their job, and be functional is gradually diminished and eventually leads to total loss of function.

The people who aren't convinced it is a real issue, have never considered the issue in the perspective of the patient. A little discomfort and natural anxiety can be accepted, however, if it becomes overwhelming and blots your daily activities and is causing a lot of stress, something must be taken care of.

That brings us to the simple inquiry. What is the point at which the sense of anxiety begin to turn into panic? The answer is quite simple. There is a change from annoyance to worry when a person's level of living is affected until it becomes inaccessible with no intervention.

In the book I refer to it gently as unsatisfactory. Why? This is because the anxiety that is caused by it affects the way you conduct yourself in other fields in such a way that it creates problems in addition of issues already affecting you. If you are unable to get out of a situation and separate it from the actions you take, you must take a step back and fix the issue. If the anxiety persists in a way that is beyond what is considered acceptable it is problems with anxiety.

The most effective way to move ahead with any concern about anxiety is to approach it with a comprehensive approach. This book's holistic strategies will consider the consequences and impacts associated with CBD oil. As a stand-alone remedy, it works for a huge segment of the population. If it is used as part of an integrated management approach and a holistic approach, it is able to be expanded to a larger population.

Holistic treatments typically focus on psychological, emotional or environmental diet, and routine considerations. There is no way to eliminate the anxiety symptoms; you must find what is causing it. If you are using CBD correctly in the most effective way it will assist to solve the issue at its base. CBD also has the capacity to alleviate symptoms and side negative effects. But why waste the potential of CBD when it could accomplish even more. But, to achieve more, you must be aware of what's happening within your body and follow the necessary steps to let CBD be more effective than the symptom-relief.

It's time to take a look at the many forms of anxiety, ranging from extreme depression to mild phobias, there are many types and levels of anxiety.

List of Anxiety Disorders

1. Phobias is an unfounded fear of an event the place or event which triggers a fearful

reaction. There are four main categories of phobias

a. The fear of sustaining a blood injury

B. Agoraphobia

C. Specific phobias and

D. Social anxiety

2. Panic Disorder is a severe anxiety disorder that is caused by bodily responses in which people are afraid of danger.

3. Generalized Anxiety includes an element in the form of "worry" which can get way out of hand. It is the most frequent form of anxiety, and results from anxiety and worry about the cause of the anxiety.

4. Obsessive Compulsive Disorder is defined by a cycle of obsessive behaviors that result in anxiety. This is then which is then followed by compulsions that reduce anxiety. There are four kinds of OCD:

I am. Symmetry obsessions

b. Sexual obsessions

C. Doing harm to other people, and

d. Contamination.

5. Body Dimorphic Disorder is a serious level of stress caused by imaginations that may trigger behavioral changes.

6. Health anxiety is characterized by intense worry regarding your health and wellbeing, which may include the fear of having a condition or dying, which can trigger behavioral modifications.

7. Post-Traumatic Stress Disorder (PTSD) can be described as the extreme anxiety and fear which is caused by an experience that was traumatized. It manifests as flashbacks, constant thoughts about the incident, repeated nightmares, as well as a tendency to avoid.

8. Habit Disorders are the habit of repetitive actions, such as cutting your nails or picking skin.

9. Sexual Difficulties: recurring difficulties in relations. They can be caused by premature ejaculation, or the erectile disorder. In women, this could comprise anorgasmia.

The majority of these problems are treated holistically through CBD as well as Cognitive Behavioral Psychotherapy.

Understanding the Basics of Anxiety

It's normal for living creatures to be afraid. This is how we safeguard ourselves. The trees and grasses also show the fear in their individual ways. This is a normal reaction. If we don't, we'll not be able trigger the"fight or flight" response or even be able to save our lives. The fight or flight response relies on an advanced neurochemical connection that controls the physiological reaction.

I'll provide the simplest explanation of anxiety and the way it is felt. In its most fundamental sense it's like having an excessive dose of caffeine. Have you ever experienced any of these? This isn't talking about the high you get from the first coffee cup, or the effects that follow from several cups. It's about that sensation that you get after having consumed the third of your cup. It's that feeling that resonates through your chest.

This sensation that you feel when you take a sensation is similar to the one it feels like when you experience an anxiety attack however, as harmless as anxiety caused by caffeine is it's uncomfortable, and you'll notice even something so simple as caffeine may trigger an feelings of anxiety. Even if it does not cause a full-blown panic attack but it's nevertheless a painful experience. The sensation is caused by chemicals. It triggers a sense of hyper-state that can cause other symptoms. The same physiological mechanism is at work for a real anxiety attack.

Distractions of this kind that is caused by caffeine, caused or stressed-induced, chemically-induced or provoked by stimuli is still distracting and distracting. In the past, I have mentioned that anxiety is an emotion that is fundamental. It's healthy when it's measured in a certain amount. What is the measurement? If this sensation prompts the person to get energized, mobilize to take action, this is a positive sign. If you're confronted with an animal that is mountain-lion, and the stress gives you strength and energy to go for a run and fight, that is a positive thing. But when that anxiety result in an incoherent and frozen condition, it's unwise, evidently.

It is important to know that we are all prone to experiencing some type of anxiety in some time throughout our lives. It is a major difficulty to recognize anxiety as normal or as an issue, and take note of the issue. Don't make the mistake of dismissing it. If you begin experiencing the tentacles of anxiety, you must observe examine, consider, and learn about what it is and what caused the anxiety. It is important to comprehend the cause and its progression over time, as well as its connection and connection to other parts in your life as well as its effects after you have let go of the triggers.

If you decide to disregard it, you'll discover that it creates more complications because the next symptom may be more severe and difficult to manage. In addition it is a missed opportunity to discover the cause and your own. If you don't take advantage of this chance the disease will be a major factor in your life. one of the ways CBD can help can be to provide you with relief from the symptoms as you determine the root of the issue.

How Much Anxiety Is Too Much?

A little anxiety can be healthy. The amount you feel anxious about is dependent on your. If you believe it's way excessive and distraction enough, then you should do something regarding it. If, on the other hand, you feel it's not a problem and gives you an advantage, then it's not necessary to act on it just make sure that it doesn't overstep the boundaries. If you're here since you're right on the line, whether or not you realize there's a problem, and you want to address the issue, your constant meditation, reflection and CBD will help you accomplish your job.

Be careful not to overreact when you see a sign of reckless conduct. This may appear to be an anxiety-provoking situation, but the increased amount of attention and concern, that may feel as anxiety, can cause you to be vigilant about the people you love and take care of your loved ones. The system keeps you and others who are around you secure through making you more cautious and puts your body in a state of consciousness.

When it reaches become too overwhelming and disruptive that it can become an issue. It can be compared to sugar, it's functional when doses are controlled. It is stimulating to the mind and can boost your energy however, if you take it overboard, it could cause permanent and unhealthy troubles. Similar to how you maintain the sugar level, it is important to maintain the frequency and intensity of your anxiety at bay. One good way to do this is to look back over your life and ask yourself questions about the frequency of your anxiety. It will assist you in analyzing what happened before you can find some level of peace with the situation.

One way to approach the anxiety issue is to view the issue as an expression of the event rather than being a self-inflicted affliction. The root of anxiety lies are in "flight-or-fight" response is real and not just fabricated mental illness, and it is important to recognize that it exists. So long as you get yourself to stop talking about it to it, it can help you in recognizing an event as what it truly is, not in being sucked into a traumatic experience or viewing everything as an imminent threat. The unknown is usually the thing that scares us most when we are scared, so if you be prepared for it and you can manage to keep it in mind, you'll have one step ahead of anxiety.

Panic Attack or Anxiety?

An attack of panic can be terrifying. This isn't only something feels inside. It involves physical and psychological signs which leave people shaken and anxious. In essence it is a heightened and compounded physical reaction to fear, anxiousness, or perhaps excitement. You read that right; it's possible to misinterpret excitement as fear and panic. Physically, both anxiety and excitement cause the same feelings - how you interpret the event which occurred and the circumstances that triggered the event, will determine where you'll go from there.

Anxiety signs can be different between individuals However, in general, anxiety manifests itself as breathing problems and chest pains, sweating and nausea - it almost it sounds like an attack on the heart, which is why the majority of patients suffering from anxiety disorders are admitted to the ER feeling they're having an attack of the heart.

From a psychological point of view From a psychological perspective, the issue is that the patient is in an increase in the level of terror. The patients are convinced they're in grave or physically threatening situation, or they've lost touch of reality.

An attack of anxiety can last from 5 to 10 minutes, or up to hours, if they are allowed to remain untreated. Its intensity can be varied also. The person may experience an intense sense of anxiety within a couple of seconds, or feel constant ache for several days. In the worst-case scenario this could result in an ongoing episode of crippling anxiety, or multiple episodes that cause short-term increases.

It is crucial to be aware of the changes that are taking place in the body of. If you're able to identify what sequence which resulted in the painful event You can then pinpoint the trigger and figure out the solution to change the cause or discover a way to stop the trigger in a way that you can be certain it will never recur.

Locating the trigger is crucial and requires some effort however, if you are able to get rid of the distracting factors that trigger you, or the root cause will appear. CBD can help in this regard in reducing background sound.

Also, you must realize that at times there's not a specific reason. The attacks that occur during sleeping can also occur when you awake with a freezing sweat. The cause could be caused from a nightmare or functioning of your unconscious mind. They are more difficult to understand and require a deeper examination.

Are Some People More Susceptible Than Others?

But it's also not just about genetics. It's all about two key factors of our mind. Human minds are made out of these elements. Genetics is the primary aspect and creates a genetic predisposition to certain traits however it's not the sole factor. The other element is physical. This is the subject of the food you consume as well as how you train as well as how much exposure you make to. Someone who has perfect genes will experience manic symptoms after exposure to mercury over the course of. It's a physical issue and is very vast. There is also the spiritual and mental aspect. A person who is exposed to pressure, stress or trauma, will continue to develop anxiety and it will manifest through as fears. The phobias will then sink into fear and anxiety.

Since no two people share the same genetic constitution as well as physical exposure and experiences in the mind so it's fairly safe to state that no individual's anxiety intensity, onset and frequency are alike.

A person's history provides a base for our current and the way one interprets this past provides the basis to be anxious about that event. Childhood memories are more profound since we are prone to keep memories in accordance with what we think of them as. If we have experienced a traumatizing incident as a child and it lingers and get worse throughout the course of the course of our childhood. Regression therapy deep is necessary to deal with events such as however, it can also be enhanced when treated using CBD.

This doesn't excuse you of the necessity to consider the implications or even if you have experienced an event of a significant nature that could cause you to feel anxious or anxious. It will make a huge positive effect on dealing with the anxiety issues.

If you don't have the confidence in their lives will most likely feel anxious as well. Even when you do have an occupation, the thought the possibility of losing it can cause anxiety in the event that you believe this isn't a safe work.

In this instance anxiety refers to the fear of possibility - and not the worry of something immediate and tangible. The issue is not being able to find satisfaction in the present as well as worrying about what could happen or not in the near future.

Myths

One common belief that contributes to anxiety is the belief that difficulties or problems are thought of as weaknesses in themselves rather than being something to be overcome and mastered. Anxiety comes from uncertainty and the thought of not knowing what will happen following or how one will manage what comes next increases the risk of being anxious. The anxiety can be reduced when one realizes that there is nothing devastating. The mistakes we make are lessons to be learned and aren't meant to be penalized. It is not fair to do not merit calamities, they are just the result of some thing. The victims of child abuse are continuously experiencing anxiety however, if they concentrate on their belief that the issue was the fault of the perpetrator rather than their fault, there's no problem that they can speak about.

It is important to note that it's not about the things that are caused by these things instead, it is about what needs to be done and what can be fixed. The truth is that there are a myriad of stories and stories that can make the water murky. Let's lay some of those out of the way And if you watch attentively, you'll start to recognize the underlying causes of myths about anxiety and will be able to use this knowledge to help you in your individual experience.

Having Anxiety Is Rare

In reality, one out of five people suffers from an anxiety disorder of some kind.

Anxiety Isn't An Illness

It's healthy to experience an appropriate degree of anxiety. However, when it turns into the disorder we described previously, it's not. The disorder can lead to impairments, and requires the treatment.

Anxiety Lasts Forever

The answer isn't. People who have anxiety-related experiences or thoughts may think that it's permanent, but this isn't the case. It is true that anxiety has a specific and consistent beginning. it's not permanent by nature, but it is rather a reactionary. When you identify the cause that is causing it, you are able to resolve the issue.

Anxiety Attack Leads To a Heart Attack

The fear of panic attacks can be terrifying because they can manifest as rapid breathing or chest pains as well as quick heartbeats. This is why it's commonplace to assume that it's an attack on the heart or that it could be a heart attack and it will, however, it's not. The root causes are different, and are psychological reactions, not physical ones.

You Can Treat Anxiety With Sedatives

The over-the-counter medicine isn't the ideal choice because they're as comprehensive as they be and will complicated issues as time passes.

This is just one of the myths individuals fall for, but they all have a common thread - which is that anxiety is not a minor issue to be dealt with just as you would treat a minor issue. But in the same way, it's not an end-all-be-all. There's a solution can be worked towards.

Signs and Symptoms of Anxiety

If you're not sure of what anxiety means, it is time to review of the signs associated with it. There are several essential elements that separate anxiety from other physical issues.

Sleep and Rest

The first step is to take a look at the patterns of your sleep. Are you able to sleep peacefully? Do you twirl and switch until it's time to wake up? Do you snore? Do you experience headaches at the beginning of your day or have muscles discomfort? Do you feel your muscles are aching after you wake up?

Headaches and muscle pains after you get up, or other symptoms which lead you to believe that you're not breathing enough oxygen while sleeping may be an indication of anxiety. This is something you should talk with your physician about. The anxiety you are experiencing could be under the surface and impacting your sleeping patterns.

Sleep is a time of anxious feelings of conscious that appear shortly before falling asleep. This happens due to the fact that you're totally at peace with your thoughts, and are not distracted by the world outside which is an time for your thoughts to focus on what might be bothering you. This is the perfect opportunity to reassess your fears and determine their real source.

Sleep disturbances are simply the excessive energized state your body enters in at the beginning of an issue. This is a sign the body that it is in good health. Imagine you're in a plane and you were asleep. If an emergency occurred at the airport or something that was urgent and growing and not yet dangerous, your body likely to shift from a state that is slumbering to one of alert. Are you able to return to sleep so the airborne emergency condition is still in the air? Absolutely not. That's the reason you shouldn't be sleeping in the night when you're dealing with an unresolved conscious or unconscious issue that isn't resolved.

The most effective way to go is to choose either or all of the following three actions.

1. Solve the real issue

2. Accept the issue both on a mental and a psychological scale.

3. Switch your focus

Social Anxiety

If you you feel the butterflies that you feel with the idea of getting to your door or getting into a crowded space or unhappy because not every Facebook friend request has been answered positively If you find like you're always stressed over every public or social circumstance, regardless of what it is, you might be suffering from a typical form of anxiety that is known as social anxiety.

Feeling Self-Conscious

Self-consciousness isn't all about ensuring that you are attractive or displaying the impression of being confident. It's about avoiding something to go wrong. this is a way of controlling the circumstances. While the basic intention and motivations behind it are good however, what it reveals is an over-evaluation of self-worth and results in a decline of confidence. In order to be able to withstand the scrutiny of those around you one must reduce the amount of attention you pay to what others consider about yourself. If you are able to overcome that problem - and it is possible to do so, then your self-consciousness will gradually disappear in an extremely short time.

Jittery Feelings

The blurred vision, the shaking hands and knees and a pounding heart are all manifestations of excessive adrenalin flowing through your body. This is the typical fighting or flight reaction, at its earliest stages, it kicks into. Because you don't know whom you have to battle or what you must do to fight, the excessive energy triggers you to physically respond. Shivers, jerks and shaking are all natural methods your body expels excessive fuel and adrenalin. It can also result by causing muscle pain as the muscles are tense and ready for intense activity. It can lead to muscle spasms, and an accumulation of lactic acid, which causes discomfort in muscles, particularly the back.

Indigestion

A different physical signification is indigestion. One of the last things your body must perform is to expend energy digestion and processing food. The body shifts its energy to muscles, brain and the senses. The body is prepared for any self-defense situations which could be triggered. Are you feeling exhausted after a dinner, or often drink an espresso after an eating out? Are you aware of how this happens? This happens when you eat a large food intake, your body goes to a state of semi-stasis where the majority of blood flows towards the stomach area in order to absorb nutrients and for the digestion of food. Siestas are a common practice for this reason. Now, when you consider it, the body, if it is fighting a battle there isn't enough capacity to focus on digestion. You notice the food going through your stomach, and identify it as an indigestion. The indigestion process throws all digestion process into chaos.

Headaches and Migraines

A state that is altered by enhanced senses and self-defense takes stress on the mind and the brain. If the body is trained to take action in situations that are alert and alert, the combination of neurotransmitters and hormones that are controlled by the primitive cortex (the brainstem) result in an increase in neuroelectric activity as well as an overloaded synapses. This causes an increase in oxygen consumption by the brain. This, consequently, raises the cerebral blood pressure in order to provide the oxygen the brain requires to function during this situation. but there's a physical limit. The heart and vessels can't supply enough oxygen which causes the brain to become suffocated and this results in suffering. Migraines and headaches occur regularly with anxiety.

Fear

It is an innate human behavior and it is controlled by the primitive brain. This is the way our ancestral ancestors reacted to dangers. If it weren't to fear, we'd have been wiped out. Imagine an antelope with no mechanism to protect itself while confronted by the predator like a lion. It is likely that you think that the lion was fed its nutrition and thus the lion lived. What happens if all antelopes die due to fearlessness? What will happen to lions in the future? The lions are being overpopulated, and aren't eating anything. They will soon also die.

Fear can be a helpful tool for social and personal reasons. It helps to keep things in check. When the brain began to develop it was in an era when life outside the body, was an easy thing. The only thing we were concerned about was being hunted and the next food source was likely to be. Our fear gave us the courage to beat our enemies and hunger provided us with the ability to pursue our quarry.

What does this have to do with have to do with CBD oil, anxiety and all of it.

CBD oil is a powerful influence on the primitive brain that includes the brainstem, as well as areas of cerebellum. Since anxiety stems from anxiety, and fears originate from the primitive portion of the brain, CBD oil is a effective tool to bring the part of our brain that is responsible for anxiety in check.

The most common definition of fear is is the result of a physiological condition that triggers by actions (combined or specific) of the different abilities of the brain (and the brain) when confronted with actual or imaginary stimulus which the individual senses (correctly or not) which can lead to imminent danger. This hazard might actually be the result of an event that is rational but it can also be an imagined event. The result is a condition of anxiety.

For a better comprehension of the fear that causes anxiety, it's important be able to dissect the definition of anxiety and identify the components of a danger as that's what's important that encapsulates the various fears and anxieties.

Elements of Hazards

Existential

The primary hazard that triggers the greatest fear is any threat to your existence either perceived or real. In an aircraft that is falling it is possible that you will feel the death of your loved ones at some point, and it is true, however when you skydive at first, you may be aware of an imminent danger. The first is true and the second can be misinterpreted. Threat detection and prevention are inherent to every living thing ranging from animals to plants as well as viruses.

Mutilation

Another common and dangerous hazard is possibility of the possibility of mutilation. Mutilation refers to the loss of limbs, or blood damage. Mutilation can also refer to things like getting bitten by dogs or getting stung by a bee. In the event of this and the resulting injuries, we can experience things like the arachnophobia.

Freedom

The number three on this listing is loss (or the possibility of losing) of liberty. The ache that comes with the loss of freedom is important - the fear of losing freedom (like the possibility of being imprisoned) is a terrifying and effective discouragement. For those who have the slightest idea of what it would be like to suffer, the pain is to be unbearable, and the anxiety can be even greater. The freedom that we enjoy isn't limited to the fear of being held in prison, it also comes with the dread of being unable to walk. A heightened sense of fear results from the fear of being confined.

Social Abandonment

Fear of being abandoned by society is the most dangerous risk. Humans are social, by nature. Collaboration brings numerous benefits as is having enjoyable. A fear of having the time to interact is crippling. Nowadays social anxiety manifests in form in the form of anxiety about having no likes or friends on social media, and then it is extended to having a good time at occasions and more. Social isolation is the precursor to demise and is an extremely powerful factor of fear. Separation anxiety is a reflection of an event.

Ego

The last, but one of the greatest dangers in our time is the end of the personal ego. Humans' egos are deep rooted in our brain and, in many instances it overrules the desire to be alive. The mind as the ego's mental model that is the body's physical. Since the mind isn't physically (the brain is, however the mind doesn't) the mind must create a frame of the body. It's similar to drawing a diagram of the mind. But when it's damaged, the mind is forced to take extremely serious notice. The mind's picture for the human body can be described as known as the self. It's a complex thing that is manifested in various ways and with different levels in all of us. The fear of losing the self is a mystery to people with a normal mind. It is one of the biggest anxiety levels.

All kinds of fears and phobia type, and kind of anxiety can be a result of one or more than one of these five risks. The severity of the danger or perception can have diverse effects on the individual.

Chapter 2: The Brain and Anxiety

For understanding anxiety, it's important be aware of a bit about the brain's evolution and the way it developed. This chapter is short to teach the basic information without diving too deeply into neuroscience and neuropharmacology.

The most important thing to know is the fact that our brain inside the cranial cavity represents working in the process (present product) of thousands of years of evolutionary progress. It is located in the brainstem which is located outside of the skull. It connects with the spine as well as the networks of nerves. The first brain was just the end of nerve endings. The entire nerve system starting from the toes to the fingers and finally to the eyelids joined to the trunk. That branch joined at the nerve-endings that create the brainstem.

Survival instincts are embedded in the brain's axons. The desire for sexual pleasure, food as well as self-preservation are encoded into this region as well. It's the human part which drives us to do what's necessary to live and spread the species.

The development of the brain has been layered, and the latest of them include elements from the neurocortex. They are the most advanced regions of the brain that be more than just binary decisions when we think of good and bad and yes or no or demons and angels. The more sophisticated we become and the more advanced we become, the more likely to understand that the world is not binary but an array of possibilities. This is only known through the advancement of the brain. However, the brain of old is still around. The brain is still there and serves a function.

Consider this for a moment Your brain that is evolved and the primitive brain share distinct interests and motives. The primitive brain wants to hunt for dinner, while your more advanced brain is more interested in going there to get his preferred cut.

Sometimes, we are caught in a battle between what our brain's primal tells us and what our more evolved brain has to say is inappropriate or socially unacceptable. The confusion that arises between what our primate brain is looking for, and the brain that evolved perceives as unsatisfactory, can lead to the state of dissonance or even confusion.

The brain's primitive part, nevertheless, is a powerful device to use. It is able to control powerful neurotransmitters that are able to entice the neocortex surrender. Consider sex for just about a second. It is a pleasure to fulfill the primary instruction is the joy of release of dopamine. Dopamine release is the transfer of fight. The neocortex becomes an opiate to dopamine after a certain thing becomes habitual regardless of whether it was initially believed by the neocortex that it was not an appropriate choice and the satisfaction of satisfying desires and the mental habits begin to establish themselves.

Over time, it's more enjoyable to examine the internal world and satisfy the needs of the primal brain as you confronted with the brain that has evolved.

How does this tie in with CBD and anxiety?

Dopamine, if it is a carrot then the brain of the primal species must also have a whip its disposal. And it certainly does. If there is a fears, relating to issues it's charged to accomplish, the primitive brain uses dopamine as well to create anxiety. Did you notice that the sensations of anxious and exuberance have the same sensation of being visceral? Since the brain stem as well as the primitive brain use chemical substances to create bouts of anxiety and fear, in addition to using the pleasure of it. The best way to manage its effects is to discover chemical substances that calm it down but without damaging it.

The ancient meditation specialists will inform that when you practice meditation and begin to renounce all the temptations that come from the flesh, it is possible to gain control over your instinctual urges. It's a way to go and can certainly be a route to take, however that's not the way we're going. What we're trying to talk about is the most direct methods to can bring the brain's primitive nature and its chemical balance and ensure that its capacity to create anxiety is greatly and profoundly diminished.

How to accomplish this appears to be it is through the use of cannabisbidiol.

The brain's primary structure is constructed upon nerve-endings, everything that your body is feeling in any remote area is reflected in the brain. If the sensation in your brain is not there then you'll not feel it. As an example, when women receive an epidural to aid in birth, they place needles between the thoracic vertebrae and inject a fluid that blocks nerve impulses. Below that point, anything cannot be transmitted back towards the brain. It completely blocks all sensations or controls from the brain.

There is no pain or controlled through, yet that is the case for all regions beneath that point and not those over it. The spinal column at different places and don't get affected. In the same way it is possible to manage your entire body by gaining access to the brain's base and administered the nerve-numbing medication in that area, you will not experience your whole body. What you feel feels the brain regardless of how strongly you believe it is located in the region which is the source of discomfort. When you shut off the signal, it cuts off sensation. Similar to that, cutting off the signal going out then you are cutting off further functions.

The brain differs than the mind. Mind is the sum total of the faculties your brain produces over the course of years. It's the experiences you have and your thoughts. This is the way that you're conditioned, and this happens in a balance between the two lower regions of your brain (lower signifying the less functions, whereas the brain's higher part that is related to art appreciation and thinking). The brain develops in time, and operates by balancing rewards and consequences. The neocortex studies current problems with the environment and conforms to what is expected and accepted our time. It is for instance, it's unacceptable in our society to consume food in a hurry or indulge in a frenzied appetite. This is why you have to learn how to behave and offer your guests the food before eating it. All of this is in your instinct. The instinct that is involved by the primitive mind, would like to consume the maximum amount of food you can and eat first, leave nothing for the next person. In time, however, we alter this urge.

This is the same with regards to how we view ourselves and the guidelines and guidelines we make for to ourselves as we age. Each of these influences our self-image and the way we portray the image we imagine of ourselves. If these things are in conflict with your instinctual self you are stressed. It is a part of anxiety created by fear.

It could be a result of an imbalance of your chemistry within the mind of your modern and primitive or the result of a misperception about how you ought to see the world. the present world. Let me explain the difference between these two. I had cats for the longest period of time when I was a child and prior to my wedding. After I got married, I needed to adjust to having an animal. That was my first exposure to dogs. I've never had one or even knew about their behavior. My husband's dog was an enormous German Shepherd and he was the most friendly dog ever. Now when he came up to me and waved his tail would cause me to get a cold. For me, as a cat's owner waving tail was a sign of trouble. For dogs however, the reverse was true. It took time, and eventually I could understand it, however my body would get into a frozen state when I noticed the tail move.

In this area of mind and psychology I realised that all it took was training, and I questioned my thinking and changed my behavior. This required a deliberate and conscious action, like saying to myself every whenever a dog walked by to not freeze in fear however, I had to keep in mind that the reason was completely different. We are afraid of things, regardless of no matter if it's right within our reach and not anxiety center gets activated, and the associated behavior is triggered.

One of the benefits of CBD that goes beyond the medical technicalities we speak about in the book - is that CBD will calm your worries from the beginning and lets you see the things as they really are. So, it gives you the chance to change the way you think about it.

Let's think about the issue the other way. It is well-known that anxiety, this feeling you experience in your body, is generated by several different things. The most important thing is that it's triggered through anxiety. Particularly, it's triggered through one of the fears which appear on the list of fears within Chapter 1. What is the reason people are afflicted with fears of jumping from a plane? It's an actual fear that people are scared that there's an opportunity that the chute isn't going to open and that they'll die. What is the reason people are afraid to stand on stage to speak? Due to anxiety of destroying their ego and the fear they'll be a sham and appear like they are less than what they appear to be. The root of all anxiety is the fear. All fear is redirected to the amygdala in the brain. It is located in the middle of the brain's primitive. I refer to it as the primitive brain as it was the first brain to evolve, and it has endured many millions of years throughout thousands of species. The brain doesn't belong to humans. The brains of cats, dogs, as well as rats, possess brains. What is different are the layers of brains which came from the evolution.

As this is not an exploration in anthropology nor neuroscience, I'll keep to the idea that the brain evolved through layers. At its top is the center of fear and the fear center is where you find the reigns. It is responsible for homeostasis. manages heart rate, manages perspiration, and in actual it is the control center for all aspects that require you to grab and sprint or hold your ground and fight confronted with danger. Therefore, it's not a surprise that if anxiety kicking in at the wrong time, there's a huge amount of dissonance in the head of your self.

The amygdala may be the cause with anxiety disorders. The research has shown that the function of the amygdala in sufferers of anxiety increases when scanned on an MRI during panic attacks. This same individual displays an amygdala that is not active when given CBD. It will be clear what causes this in Chapter 3.

Chapter 3: Cannabidiol

If you're not aware of that, CBD stands for Cannabidiol. It comes from hemp plants and in the past, CBD was an important source of contention within the legislative world. It was a banned drug and is still in several states, however worldwide, it's beginning to gain acceptance as a medicine instead of a hallucinogenic drug or a drug that is addictive. Its name Cannabis is also known as Marijuana is the name given to the plant the substance comes from, has also earned an image, though it is not well-known. Due to these two factors the use and acceptance of the oil has been gradual, however it is now getting the respect it merits.

The plant of cannabis has yielded so far 113 distinct chemicals - known as cannabinoids. Two cannabinoids you might have heard about comprise Cannabidiol (CBD) as well as Tetrahydrocannabinol (THC). They are among the most well-known among the various cannabinoids that are found in cannabis.

Contraindications

Before we get started, it's important to know that not everybody could benefit from CBD. If you're taking specific kinds of medications, or for specific sorts of diseases and conditions, you should know that CBD is something that has to be examined by a medical professional. Here are some typical contraindications to CBD.

Steroids

HMG CoA reeducates inhibitors

Calcium channel blockers

Antihistamines

Prokinetics

HIV antivirals

Immune modulators

Benzodiazepines

Anti-arrhythmic

Antibiotics

Anesthetics

Anti-psychotics

Anti-depressants

Anti-epileptics

Beta-blockers

PPIs

NSAIDs

Angiotensin II blockers

Hypoglycemic drugs for oral use

Sulfonylureas

Please read this if you are currently or were a victim of serious illnesses such as COPD epilepsy, COPD or cancer, in which case CBD or THC might have an excellent medical possibilities, it is important to discuss this with your doctor to determine the way CBD can interact with your existing medication.

CBD Source

If you're using CBD oil, research and study behind its effects will not be useful when the oil is affected by contamination or has been diluted. The oil could also be inadequately manufactured. People who are passionate about making the oils and tinctures themselves However, the best solution is to buy quality CBD oil from a reliable CBD vendor.

Though I'm not a fan of each one but I'll provide you with a some names of those to consider before deciding on where to buy CBD oil.

NuLeaf Naturals

Pure Spectrum

Receptra Naturals

Endoca

CW Botanicals

Bluebird Botanicals

Green Garden Gold

Imbue Botanicals

Isodiol

Cannadiol

Cannabinoids and How They Work

Cannabinoids which are made from plants are usually identified by their phytocannabinoids. CBD as along with THC are phytocannabinoids since they're the cannabinoids which come directly from plants, they aren't derived inside your body, or from any other source or alternative source.

Cannabinoids influence receptors in the family of cannabinoid that is found in the central nervous system and also in the peripheral nervous network. They change the patterns and amount of neurotransmitters released. This is the way in which the limbic system (the most ancient part of the brain) is accountable for the cognitive process of the neocortex.

THC could be involved in the release and the production of dopamine which is the neurotransmitter we have discussed in our previous chapter. Dopamine is a neurotransmitter that plays an important role in the mechanism of reward and punishment which brains. Dopamine release triggers feelings of joy across the entire body. When you do something, the brain's primitive portion approves that the brain's release of dopamine. Following a few occasions, the neocortex becomes aware that when it executes what the limbic system wants the reward will be given and then the behavior develops. It was shown in the preceding chapter. In the next chapter, THC performs the same function similar thing as THC however, it gives people the pleasure of energy and a sensation that is intense. However, it does not require acquiescence to the brain's directives.

Central nervous system, as well as peripheral nerves originate at the level of the brain. It continues to move through the spinal column and on to every other area of the body. This was discussed earlier in this section. The receptors situated near the ends of nerves are called cannabinoid receptors. The whole system is often referred to by the term endocannabinoid system. Two receptors comprise the ones which we'll study during this research namely CB1 in addition to CB2.

CB1 - Cannabinoid Receptors Type 1

CB1 can be present in the brain as well as throughout the nervous network. They are situated in the basal nuclei in the limbic system and hippocampus and also in the cerebellum of the cerebral cortex. They are as well found to have significant concentration throughout reproductive organs for both genders.

CB1 Lowers Anxiety and Stress

Based on studies of the mice, it was discovered that those who do not have CB1 receptors, don't have an amygdala that is larger and have more anxiousness. This is an important factor in the management of anxiety, especially when you are stressed.

Remember that CB1 is present at higher levels in the nerve system's central region, however it is greater in the hippocampus as well as the amygdala that is found within the cerebral cortex. These are important areas in the control of emotional and memory. In addition it is believed that they could have a role in ADHD as well as emotional regulation anxiety problems and mental health problems.

CB1 receptors also have been proven to influence serotonin manufacturing (this contributes to the dopamine release procedure we discussed previously.)

Prefrontal Cortex

The infusion of cannabis-based cannabinoids into the system is thought to have an impact on the prefrontal brain, and the introduction of these cannabinoids has been believed to boost the activity of the frontal cortex while simultaneously stimulating the amygdala. Research regarding anxiety has shown that it has been linked to reduced activities in the prefrontal cortex as well as increased activity within the amygdala. Contrary to this, and the most balancing element, is cortisol. It is found to be with higher levels in individuals that are not able to fight anxiety.

Cannabinoid receptors have been inhibited by medications.

for studies of people who have no mental health issues there was a 300 percent more anxiety-related symptoms was discovered when the participants had a screening with an anti-cannabinoid medication. There was an additional report that indicated there increased degree for depression. This decreased when the drug was removed from the treatment with anti-cannabinoid. In addition there was evidence through a myriad of research studies that CB1 blocking drugs made people to look less positive.

CB1 and Post Traumatic Stress Disorder (PTSD)

A number of studies revealed that evidence suggests the endocannabinoid system in the human body is an important part in regulating stress, anxiety and overall wellbeing.

The research has revealed that the psychological effects of stress influence the levels of Anandamide in the brain. Anandamide is a neurotransmitter created in the brain. It's attached to CB1. When everything is functioning as planned The brain releases this neurotransmitter, ensuring that there's no stress. In stressful situations, it releases neurotransmitters and the sufferers begin feeling the negative side effects of stress. Stress may reduce levels of anandamide within the limbic area. The levels decreased will return to normal in the space of 24 hours after the stress event was over. The results of research have revealed research that the reduction in Anandamide directly affects the amount of the cortisol produced in stressful situations.

In the event that when you realize that it's possible that the CB1 receptor isn't functioning or is damaged, there could rise the anxieties. It is obvious that there is an underlying reduction in the capacity to control anxiousness. It also causes chain reactions that involve the pituitary gland and hypothalamus and also the adrenal gland which is responsible for cortisol production.

When patients were exposed to cannabinoids in particular the prefrontal cortex, neuron were activated dramatically, followed by a decrease of GABA release. Also, it reduced GABA release, and excitability in the amygdala.

GABA (Gamma-Aminobutyric acid, also known as GABA is also known as GABA (g-aminobutyric acids) can be defined as a neurotransmitter and the principal inhibitor of Central Nervous System in human beings. Its main role is to lower the excitability of neurons in the nerve system.

The results of clinical trials show that CB1 receptors have been proven to exhibit tangible effects by using activators, such as CBD in treating PTSD and general anxiety disorder. While appealing as it might sound, make sure you are aware of the fact that drinking regularly and often of marijuana has been shown to result in a decline in performance of the amygdala situations of stress. It has been proven that people suffering from PTSD are positive for an incredibly decreased level of anandamide. In addition, they show a significant decrease in the 2-AG. Further, it was proven that the levels are in line with the ones experienced by those suffering from trauma however, they do not experience post-traumatic anxiety.

2-AG, or 2-Arachidonoylglycerol, is an endocannabinoid (a cannabinoid that is produced by the body). It's an activater for CB1 and CB1 as well as CB2 receptors. 2AG is an a fatty acid-based molecules.

In rodents less CB1 receptors exhibit a higher frequency and an increased amygdala. It is known as the center of anxiety. It is an opportunity to understand how the endocannabinoid process inside the body plays an important function in stress, anxiety and stress.

CB2 - Cannabinoid Receptors Type II

It was initially believed that CB1 was the only receptor in the body. CB1 was the most important that had endocannabinoid receptors present in the human body. This has been disproved for quite some time and CB2 is now a recognized and validated receptor in the body too.

Also, it was discovered that CB2 isn't only found in very high levels in the brain, but throughout the immune system, as it is in every single node within the immune system. These include the tonsils, thalamus, as well as the spleen. It is crucial to remember that these are key production sites for Cytokines. The study also found CB2 receptors inside different immune cells across the body, including monocytes.

Yet, regardless of how large they may be however, the highest concentration of CB2 receptors is found inside the hypothalamus. This is in the prefrontal cortex, the brainstem the basal Ganglia as well as the microglia (a kind of immune system cells only found in the brain). In addition, since they can be found in the brain. CB2 receptors may also be found in the stomach as well as inside the intestinal tract. They are able to inhibit inflammation. This is the reason CB2 is a feasible alternative for treating intestinal inflammation that originates from the digestive tract including Crohn's Disease.

Mastocytes, also referred to in the field of mast cells form them an essential part of the immunity systems. In response to stimulation, they generate and release histamine, heparin as well as other compounds. The CB2 receptors of mastocytes control their functionality and influence their function. This has an immediate impact on how often and how much histamine and histamine that is released to our body.

CB2 can also be a inhibitor of activation and T-cell proliferation. For patients with Alzheimer's disease the neuron's function is diminished due to the formation plaque. The plaque is formed of beta-amyloid proteins. The role CB2 has in this regard is essential because they're capable of activating macrophages (cells that kill other cells) in addition to destroying the plaque which interferes with the normal firing process of neurons. It is evident that activation CB2 receptors may be used in the fight against Alzheimer's.

The most shocking results of the studies conducted in the various medical fields that encompass a wide range of disciplines, is the fact that almost all illnesses that affect our body are characterized by an increase in the level of the endocannabinoid. Whatever the reason, be it mental or digestive, neurologic, endocrine or dermatological, they all are likely to have solutions in the area of CB2 activation and control. There is some evidence suggesting that CB2 receptors could be activated in order to reduce the chance of becoming addicted to cocaine.

What Does CBD do Exactly?

CBD doesn't have any psychoactive properties similar to its close relative THC. Actually, CBD is able to minimize the negative effects caused by THC in some degree, and, when combined with, CBD acts as a alternative to THC in order to give the user the euphoria that the user experiences.

CBD is a receptor for CBD connects to CB1 in addition to the CB2 receptors inside the human body. CBD functions, as we have mentioned in the past, to act as an antagonist for THC and antagonists to cannabinoid. This is the reason why CBD an effective tool in battling the harmful impacts of the other cannabinoids. This is an actual truth that indicates that CBD gives us benefits of cannabinoids but without the psychoactive impact of THC or one other of the hundreds of other constituents that make up cannabis.

The research has shown that CBD can also have an impact on serotonin and Adenosine, along with glycine levels (to control the body's temperature and being able to sense the effects of heat on discomfort). When there's a fire that results in injury, CBD could be utilized to alleviate the burning sensation.

CBD may also possess an effective antidepressant effect. It was found that CBD could help in activating the serotonin receptor 5-HT1A, which is thought to cause antidepressant effect. The receptor is also involved in influencing the perception of pain, appetite, anxiety as well as the addiction process.

Furthermore the research suggests that CBD aids in reducing the growth of cancerous cells and aids in restoring bone through inhibiting the GPR55-mediated signaling.

GPR55 is the dominant pathway for signaling within the brain that is linked to controlling blood pressure, managing bone density, as well as the growth of cancerous cells.

Medical Application

CBD and CBD oil and, in turn CBD oil, have these benefits:

Antiemetic (reduces nausea and vomiting)

* Anticonvulsant (suppresses seizure activity)

*Antipsychotic (combats psychosis related disorder)

*Anti-inflammatory (combats inflammation-related diseases)

* Antioxidant (combats neurodegenerative disorders

* Anxiolytic/antidepressant (combats anxiety and depression disorders)

The aspect we're attracted to about this book is its Antipsychotic and Antidepressant qualities.

CBD as an Antipsychotic/Antidepressant

Cannabis can trigger severe psychotic episodes when it is consumed in large quantities or under certain conditions. Studies have found that smoking marijuana can increase chances of suffering from persistent psychosis in individuals with certain genetic risk factors.

It's fascinating to note the fact the results of clinical research that showed THC may be the catalyst of these outcomes. This is the reason why CBD is thought to be a good choice. CBD could counteract the effects of psychoactive substances by being the antipsychotic. That makes CBD an efficient method to reduce the dosages of psychoactive effects of THC.

Many studies carried out by medical researchers have recently included those with psychotic symptoms like those who are suffering from schizophrenia. They involved were performed using CBD. The positive results were seen.

Additionally, there are studies on those who suffer from Parkinson's disease. These patients also had positive results after treatment with CBD. However, the method is not over, however additional clinical trials will be required to evaluate the efficacy of CBD as well as its negative effects for patients with schizophrenia as well as different types of psychosis.

CBD is proved by research conducted on animal models that CBD is able to reduce stress and also lower it due to the diminution of behavioral and physiological symptoms related to stress and anxiety. It is an ideal indication for research. There are some Human Clinical and lab trials which have proven that CBD is useful and efficient.

For studies on chronic post-traumatic disorder resulting from stress CBD has proven that CBD may increase the capability of patients to erase the traumatic memories that accompany memories. The anxiety-reducing effects of CBD were evident by the activation of the serotonin receptor 1. It is essential to continue conducting research on this subject, however the evidence we've seen to date is to be positive.

The various combination used in lab tests and tests, the most efficient outcomes were obtained by using THC along in conjunction with CBD. As you might recall, CBD counteracts many of the negative side effects caused by THC and also its psychoactive effects.

Researchers have observed positive outcomes by using synthesized cannabinoids. One such synthetic can be JWH-133. This is a cannabinoid molecule found by J.W.Huffman. It is an molecule that is able to attach specifically to CB2 receptors. Research has demonstrated that it can be used to reduce the formation of markers for cognitive impairment, and also to lower inflammation among Alzheimer sufferers.

Side Effects

It's crucial to remember that, even though it's much more safe than its cousin THC drug there are limitations on the amount of THC you're allowed to consume and also the frequency you can use the drug. In the earlier times, we have discussed being immune to the effects of it, however, in this piece the side effects we'll discuss are those that may make you vulnerable by doses that are over the limit of dosage to use on a daily basis in conjunction with other supplements that are contraindicated, or when it is taken in conjunction under certain situations. Like any other medication, CBD is essential to be aware about how you take CBD.

Most commonly reported negative side effect is dry mouth. Be aware that you should drink plenty of water before the time when your first CBD dose is given. This will help ease the discomfort.

The effect is apparent of a lower blood pressure. CBD acts as a vasodilator. This means it's capable of dilation of blood vessels and, as a result, lowers the pressure in the blood. If you're taking blood pressure medication which isn't working, this could be a problem and that's the reason we've added CBD in chapter 3.

It is also possible to be dizzy and this could result from the vasodilation issue that was previously mentioned. If you notice a decrease in pressure within the blood vessels, it reduces circulation of oxygen into different parts of your body, including your cerebrum. If you're susceptible to experiencing the sensation of being lightheaded, consult your physician about your frequency of feeling lightheaded. might be feeling. This is an opportunity to develop into Drowsiness.

When you're pregnancy and concerns about birth There isn't enough information and studies available to determine the effects it has on the baby and mother. Again, talk to your obstetrician and doctor as well. It is identical if breastfeeding. Anything you consume can be found in the milk you give your baby, and that's why it's important to not make use of CBD when breastfeeding.

The CBD Institute has repeatedly stated that CBD may have psychotropic effects. There have been a handful of instances of individuals who are very sensitive, which are verified. There could be many factors that cause this like sensitiveness to the CBD chemical, or insufficient distillation techniques or techniques for tincturing. For this reason, purchase CBD from trustworthy and reliable suppliers.

Chapter 4: CBD Oil and Anxiety

What we've presented is a huge subject. It covers the two most important research and clinical fields like the neuroscience field and Pharmacology. There's plenty to learn, however the most important thing to remember is it's two disciplines.

There are two methods to handle anxiety. The first will make it easier to manage the process. It starts with the thoughts you make will be processed by your brain's neurocortex. It is then perceived by your brain. How you interpret is in relation to the relation between you and the opponent will be determined in this stage. The brain's fear centers of your brain are activated into action, and create a condition of alertness that is in an effort to defend yourself against any danger.

However, it is an ideal scenario. If you're in a healthy state of mind and keep a steady consciousness, how you look at things and the way you view it will inform your experience and prompt what reaction you should take. If, but you're experiencing anxiety that's too intense, the perception of your body can be read as a fear reaction and your fear response is activated.

The layer below is as well. This layer is physical in contrast to the psychological layer that was first. Chemically, in the event that you suffer from the hyperactive center of fear or an increased amygdala (which is where you find anxiety) and even when the perception is correct and there's nothing you need to worry regarding, your anxiety centre can override your impression and make you feel like the body itself alerts you to the fact that you are in danger. It could increase hair growth at the neck's nape or intense anxiety attacks.

The treatment of anxiety disorders can be accomplished using one of two strategies and is advised using both. The other is that you could enhance and reflect your personal. Also, it is the release of cannabinoids from the body. If you're suffering from low levels of these substances, your receptors become less active. In addition, when you make the use of CBD you are getting the same chemical your body produces to ensure the normalization of the body's psychological system.

The other alternative is to eat supplements that are external - they're the phytocannabinoids that we've discussed. Although there are THC cannabinoids and CBD cannabinoids. But, it is certain we're not discussing THC. But, CBD however, on contrary has shown to provide an extremely promising result for resolving the issues.

However, the best method to reduce anxiety is to use CBD oil. It can help soothe your nerves, according to the phrase that you should wait until you're in a position to determine. You can then think about looking into the matter and removing anxiety and worries is much more straightforward rather than in the midst of a crisis or in the midst of a situation. CBD oil is taken by many as CBD oil, which can offer you an increase of neurotransmitters. This can enable you to be relaxed in order to evaluate the situation with a clear mind and enjoy the peace in the future when you'll need it.

For someone who has promoted CBD to help with anxiety It's the right time to think about things that aren't beneficial. CBD does not fit everyone. If you encounter someone who says contrary to what they say, they may not give you the full truth.

CBD is also harmful in the event of misuse CBD when you misuse it. What is the best way to use CBD especially because CBD does not have the psychoactive properties of a psychoactive ingredient Many people use CBD seeking a quick answer to the anxiety concerns. Take note that CBD doses can provide instant relief for a short period duration, due to phytocannabinoids being released which are doing what they are supposed to do. This is like playing with the game. You're fine if you're trying it for confidence that you can solve your issue and not to continue repeating the same routine.

CBD is one of the substances which is often hyped. Even if you do not notice any positive outcomes, there's a chance that CBD may be excessively used. Be aware that it's not an intoxicant, but it is designed to release neurotransmitters that the body might not be ready or not be able to let go of.

It's crucial to be aware that your mind keeps track of everything you do. Once your mind starts to realise that it is able to quickly stop an issue that is occurring, it will need it to be constantly on the lookout for ways to make sure you're capable of blocking any issue. What's likely occur is instead of initiating the"fight or fight" response, no matter if it's not the right reaction will be to search for

CBD. Your brain and body are living, advanced things. Try not to think about it for the rest throughout your lifetime.

As we have explained in this article, CBD is a powerful aid in relieving anxiety, whether it's general anxiety or a specific anxious. It's your option to use CBD to ease your anxiety, and not take it for a treatment.

Chapter 5: The Genesis of CBD Oil

Cannabis is an incredibly popular trend. At one time, it was looked at as a thing only taken by hippies or snooty students with bongs hidden beneath their beds.

However, there are various reasons cannabis is making its place in the world of medicine but, sadly cannabis isn't utilized in medical treatment in the same way similar to other prescription drugs.

Cannabis has been found to be as a treatment option rather than at the "needs to be treated" side of the spectrum.

The element of cannabis that deserves to be praised for is CBD which is one of many elements of marijuana. After extraction, CBD doesn't possess any psychoactive effects.

This is a good choice for all users to consider. It's 100% pure (even when extracted) And even it's safe for children. World Health Organization has given it a thumbs up, declaring that it's safe and has none side effects that you need to be concerned about (Geneva 2018, 2018).

Simply put, it's all that's needed to a natural, healthful, holistic solution which is quite distinct from typical chemical-based medications available currently available.

Although cannabis itself may produce a smokey buzz and fog, CBD is a whole completely different beast.

The CBD/THC/cannabis debate is an enigma. This article will attempt to make sense of it by looking into the background of the plant, its extraction process, as well as the amazing element, so that you can get an idea about what exactly you're getting in the form of CBD oil.

The History of Cannabis

Cannabis has been around for longer than we think. The very first variety of cannabis,

Cannabis Sativa, has been grown for thousands of years.

The nature of this plant to have been cultivated and utilized over thousands of years can be a sign of its value. The past was a time when plant species were cultivated to provide food and medicinal purposes, however, it was only a few years later that the idea of growing for recreation become popular.

In the present, CBD is being used in a variety of ways, from relaxing to alleviating symptoms for both pets and humans.

China

Archaeologists have discovered numerous signs that hemp was used the 1122nd year of BC in evidence by fragments of hemp fabric found that were found in the antiquated Chinese burial chambers. Hemp paper fragments as well as hemp bowstrings have been discovered.

The Chinese Emperor, Shen-Nung (c.2700 BC), is believed to have been the first person to utilize cannabis in order to benefit from its healing properties. Actually, he's considered to be the founder of Chinese Medicine, and after conducting tests on poisons, herbs, as well as antidotes, created a medical dictionary, known as the Pen Ts'ao. In the book, we see cannabis, also known as "ma" listed as an efficient medicine (Hou 1977).

Based on the experience of Shen-Nung the plant, Chinese used it for a while as a treatment for menstrual issues, gout, arthritis as well as constipation and memory issues.

Around the early 2nd century AD an important Chinese surgeon realized the benefits of cannabis as a pain reliever. He started combining cannabis (ma) along with win (yo) in order to develop a poultice (ma-yo) that he put on during surgery to ease the discomfort of the patient (Gumbiner 2011).

India

India also has an extensive history of connection to cannabis. The cannabis' first mention is in one of the most sacred Hindu texts known as the Vedas dating from around 2000 BC.

According to Vedic traditions the cannabis plant was among five plants that were sacred, and is a healer that brought joy, eased anxiety and gave us confidence.

Cannabis is frequently referred to as an alcohol in Indian texts. It is mixing with different spices and herbs to make it into a savoury liquid. Also, it can be consumed in tiny balls, paired with milk or smoke with a pipe for the basis of a group activity.

In the early 1890s, the British began to be concerned by the massive consumption of cannabis, also known as bhang in India The

British commissioned research into the preparation, cultivation and the social and moral impact of this substance.

Following four years of research and collation, their results showed that there was not a need to restrict the usage of this herb since it did not show any evidence of having any negative effects to anyone in anyway (Caine 1893).

It is still widely used even in everyday routine and during religious ceremonies. In some areas of the nation you can purchase it in a legal manner from street sellers.

United Kingdom

The first time the world really started to recognize cannabis for its medicinal properties around 1839 when William Brook O'Shaughnessy published a journal that detailed his research in the Calcutta institution studying its effects on the body (Mukherjee 2017, 2017).

Just a little over 100 years later, around the year 1940 Robert S. Cahn who was an British chemical scientist, discovered the chemical structure that is Cannabinol (CBN).

America

In the same period as the discovery of Cahn, American chemical chemist Roger Adams made two significant advancements in the field of cannabis. He discovered the first cannabis-derived cannabinoid Cannabidiol (CBD) as well as was also the one responsible in the discovery that of Tetrahydrocannabinol (THC).

Hemp was used since before the Revolution it was utilized for making cloth, paper rope, and paper.

In the early 20th century, hemp was first used for psychoactive purposes. Hemp and marijuana were both prohibited, and as the effort to reduce cultivation and usage in the country, the government passed the Marihuana Tax Act of 1937 which stated that only hemp which was recognized and taxed by authorities would be allowed.

After this, it was when Adams and his colleagues discovered their groundbreaking discovery, which was recognized from the Dr. Walter Loewe soon thereafter. He conducted tests on CBD as well as THC in rabbits concluding that THC was a stimulant as well as CBD did not have any beneficial properties.

It wasn't until the early 1960s in the 1960s that Israeli researcher Raphael Mechoulam and his team were keenly studying CBD and started to realize the health benefits of CBD.

As of now, the medical authorities within the US government put cannabis into the same class of highly toxic, addictive drugs including heroin and LSD.

With this distinction, the in-depth investigation became more challenging. An incredibly small number of scientists continued to research cannabis however, they made another breakthrough in the year 1992 when Mechoulam, William Devane, and Lumir Hanus were able to identify two important cannabinoids naturally produced by the body of a human.

These breakthroughs led to the development of the endocannabinoid process and a realization that our bodies were made to respond to cannabinoids like CBD as well as THC.

The trend for cannabis only started to grow in the early 2000s, with numerous hemp-related and CBD-related laws that were passed over the last few times.

The Legal Struggle

Cannabis was smuggled under the rug throughout the decades, and it remained a prohibited drug until quite recently.

It's important to remember that laws differ across different nations, as well as diverse laws regarding the cannabis plant as well as

CBD (cannabidiol) in recreational usage as well as medicinal uses.

Some countries place limitations regarding cannabis use as a recreational substance. CBD and medicinal cannabis are becoming more popular, even though they are still illegal in numerous nations across the globe.

The countries where both medical and recreational cannabis is legally available (with certain restrictions) comprise Uruguay, South Africa, Georgia and Canada.

Some countries have chosen to not criminalize cannabis for recreational use and have restrictions specific to the specific region. This includes Antigua and Barbuda, Argentina, Austria, Australia, Belgium, Belize, Bermuda, Bolivia, Chile, Colombia, Costa Rica, Croatia, Czech Republic, Ecuador, Estonia, Israel, Italy, Jamaica, Luxembourg, Malta, Mexico, Moldova and Moldova, the Netherlands, Paraguay, Peru, Portugal, Saint Kitts and Nevis, Saint Vincent and the Grenadines, Slovenia, Spain, Switzerland, Trinidad and Tobago, and several regions in the USA.

Medical cannabis is completely legal throughout Argentina, Australia, Barbados, Bermuda, Brazil (for those who have exhausted all other possibilities), Canada, Chile, Colombia, Croatia, Cyprus, Czech Republic, Denmark, Ecuador, Finland (with the approval of a license), Georgia, Germany (for people who've exhausted their other alternatives), Greece, Ireland, Israel, Italy, Jamaica, Lebanon, Lithuania, Luxembourg, Malawi, Malta, Mexico (THC content lower than 1percent) and Mexico, the Netherlands, New Zealand, North Macedonia, Norway, Pakistan (CBD only), Poland, Portugal, Romania (THC content below 0.2 percent), Saint Vincent and the Grenadines, San Marino, Slovenia, South Africa, Spain (limited), Sri Lanka, Switzerland, Thailand, Turkey, United Kingdom (when recommended by a qualified specialist), Uruguay, Vanuatu, Zambia, and Zimbabwe.

United States

Within the United States, medicinal cannabis is permitted in all the states of 45, 4 territories in addition to four territories, and the District of Columbia. However, it is illegal on the federal level.

It is legal to use for recreational purposes (with limitations) in several states. The use of marijuana for any purpose was prohibited across every state.

The first demonstration against the ban on cannabis was in the year 1964 when Lowell Eggemeier lit a joint at the San Francisco Hall of Justice and then demanded that he be detained. The incident sparked the uprising against marijuana laws.

In the wake of in the year 1970's Controlled Substances Act, in the 1970s, when cannabis was declared illegal on every level The movement to legalize cannabis began to take off. Oregon is the state that was first in America to declare legal in 1973. It was followed by Nebraska in the year 1978.

The presidency of Jimmy Carter in 1976 was thought to be a catalyst for moving it ahead, given that he had spoken highly in support of decriminalization. However, at the conclusion in the 1970s He had completely turned to the other side strongly urging that it remain illegal.

1981 was the year of Ronald Reagan taking over the presidency. Reagan along with the first lady together with a variety of concerned parents organizations, stopped the effort to legalize marijuana.

In the past two decades, the law was not enacted during the battle to legally legalize the use of cannabis, up until the year 2001 which was the year that Nevada has been decrimalized. The states of 16 have now removed cannabis from the criminal justice system, and nine states are making a move towards and legally allowing marijuana.

The legalization fight for recreational marijuana ended up winning in two states: Washington in Washington and Colorado, in 2012. In the years since, 16 jurisdictions have approved cannabis usage and most include cultivation, as well as distribution.

Difference Between CBD and THC

There's a significant distinction among CBD (cannabidiol) as well as cannabis. Though many people utilize cannabis to treat many ailments (and it is effective), CBD is slightly distinct.

Cannabis is a type of plant. It can be dried and smoke it, or use it to make tea leaves or bake using cannabis.

Cannabis plants contain more than 100 elements. The most widely known components are known as phytocannabinoids which contain two of the most popular name: CBD and THC.

CBD is therefore only a small portion of cannabis (and as such, so is THC).

What's the major differences in CBD and THC and what's the reason this have any significance?

CBD VS THC

CBD (cannabidiol) and THC (tetrahydrocannabinol) are entirely different components of the cannabis plant.

Consider it in terms of white and red blood cells. They're two distinct components of blood with various roles that they play but they're both in the same place the blood.

It's the same when it comes to CBD as well as THC. Both are quite different in the way they affect that they exert for the human body however, they're all one thing: the cannabis plant.

Let's start by introducing THC.

In its entirety, THC doesn't do much. When you combine it with the other components present in cannabis, and you'll find it's got amazing properties that help fight sleepiness, increase appetite, decrease anxiety and ease discomfort.

Yes, it gets you high.

THC is an euphoric substance. It is a compound that can bring extreme joy and the sensation of having your head being suspended in cloud. However, in a few instances, it may cause the opposite effect and stir an anxiety-like feeling.

A significant portion of how people or recreational users respond to THC depends on the way they feel at that present.

And now, let's move on to CBD.

People who want to enjoy the benefits of cannabis, but not the effects of a high could do it with CBD. CBD is a great option to use in many methods, such as in edibles, tinctures, teas and even vapes.

The research suggests that CBD helps in decreasing inflammation, reducing seizures, relieving the symptoms of depression and anxiety as well as improving skin problems and treating cancer. It also helps in reducing chronic pain, and reducing degenerative illnesses.

It is not yet clear as the effects it has on several of these fields However, preliminary evidence suggests its results are genuine and in some instances astonishing.

Further research has shown that CBD as well as THC are both able to produce the strongest effects when they are used in conjunction. This is referred to as"the effect of entourage" (Russo 2011,).

Difference Between Hemp and Marijuana

As we've explained, the phrase "cannabis" refers to a plant. For more precise definition it is an entire species of plants and there exist two variations from that species, cannabis and hemp.

The distinction is straightforward The difference is that marijuana is rich in THC and contains moderate levels of CBD and CBD, whereas hemp is a great source of CBD and has a low amount of THC.

If you're looking for a high cannabis is the drug you should go with. If you're looking for positive health effects, hemp is ideal for those who want to get healthy.

Contrary to what many believe it isn't necessarily bad for anyone. The consumption of it as either a tincture or the form of an edible can cause feeling of euphoria, but it has advantages of its own. the modest concentration of CBD is a good addition to the advantages.

Marijuana smoking can cause adverse unwanted side effects. However, they are mostly due to the smoke itself and not the actual substance (American Chemical Society 2007, 2007).

The health benefits associated with using marijuana for medical purposes are being studied, however the first findings suggest that the effect of entourage is powerful, provided you are able to take the effects of the high.

Hemp plants are a little just 0.3 percentage THC. Even with their greater CBD quantity, it is still many hemp plants for the production of CBD oil or tinctures. If you're looking to reap the health advantages of CBD with the safety of THC CBD, hemp-based products are the best way to take.

It is important to remember that hemp oil as well as CBD oil aren't identical. When you're seeking CBD oil or hemp is crucial to ensure that the seller is honest about the source of their product and the process of making it.

Hemp is a bioaccumulator. It soaks up everything and anything it comes into contact with, and if it is grown in soils that have been treated using pesticides, the plant can be polluted. Be sure to look for a Certification of Analysis before purchasing (Astorino, 2018,). It will show that the product has evaluated by a third party and is deemed to be genuine.

How CBD Oil Is Made

Three steps are involved in the creation of CBD oil:

* Extraction of CBD from the plant. CBD out of the cannabis

* Getting rid of the components that are not needed

* Add an oil carrier

We'll go over each step a little greater detail.

Extraction Methods

After the kind of plant is decided on (hemp or marijuana) is the time to extract CBD from the plant. There are three different ways that extract CBD from cannabis.

* Steam-Based Extraction Methods

* Solvent-Based Extraction Methods

* CO2 Extraction Steam-Based Extraction

Steam extraction is among the oldest method. It takes a substantial amount of hemp in order to create only a tiny quantity of CBD however, it could be a risky process. It is difficult to determine the exact amount of CBD which is why it can also be easy to get it incorrect.

The method requires three distinct flasks. The first flask is filled with boiling water. It is connected to one of the glass flasks that houses Cannabis plants. Above that, there is what's known as"the "condenser tube", which is where the finished product gets recollected.

When the water is boiling, the steam is brought into contact with the plants and dissociating CBD from CBD via oil and vapors. The vapors that rise up and are absorbed by the condenser tube. There, they are separated in water and oil. The mixture is then decanted in order to separate the CBD from its pure CBD.

Solvent-Based Extraction

The process works similarly with steam-based extraction. It is different in that the steam-based method uses water, this technique employs the solvent of your choice.

A solvent is a chemical which dissolves various other compounds. After this, what's left is referred to as a solution as well as the solvent that's formed disappears leaving the product that is left behind, CBD.

Most commonly-used solvents comprise hydrocarbon solvents (butane propane, butane, petroleum) as well as natural solvents (ethanol or olive oil).

The solvents of hydrocarbons are a danger due to the fact that the residue created by these chemicals can be harmful and can increase the chance of developing cancer as well as other health hazards.

Natural solvents can also pose issues, though they're much less harmful than hydrocarbons. If you use one of these chemicals the chlorophyll is expelled from the plants, leading to an unpleasant taste. It is possible to remedy this by using a quality oil, or by turning the CBD into a food.

Another issue in the case of natural solvents is they don't completely evaporate which means that there is less CBD left within the solution. This is more as compared to other techniques.

CO2 Extraction

CO2 extraction can be described as the most efficient cheap, efficient, and clean method of obtaining CBD. Also, it's fairly consistent with the amount of CBD that it produces, which means you'll receive the exact amount of CBD for the same plant matter every single time.

The method employs a special device that is able to compress carbon dioxide till it is in an extremely cold liquid state. The process of passing the plant through the liquid, it removes CBD.

It's a method that is widely used that is affordable and provides a significant quantity of CBD it does not leave any residue behind that could harm environmental protection than all the other options.

Removal of Unwanted Compounds

What is extracted from the plant is deemed as "full-spectrum" CBD. This means that it contains lots of elements from the cannabis plant and not only CBD.

If producers want to take out other components, additional processes are needed. Following further processing, the final product will be a full spectrum, broad-spectrum or an separated CBD extract.

Adding a Carrier Oil

The final step is to mix the CBD extract with carrier oil. What is the reason for an oil? It is because they permit producers to dilute their mixture in the amount that is required as well as assist your body absorb oil quicker.

Naturally, they'll also enhance flavor! Most commonly-used oils are coconut oil, MCT oil as well as hemp seed oil.

When these processes have been done, a third-party test is essential (Roger 2020). This is the reason why an Certificate of Analysis is important since it indicates this product has been tested to be of good quality.

Different Strengths and Concentrations of CBD Oils

There are many different kinds of CBD oil. CBD oil is made equal and that's what makes it so effective in treating many ailments efficiently.

Manufacturers distill CBD extract into oil until it is at the concentration that they want. After extraction it is able to produce CBD usually is 99 percent pure. It requires some distillation before it is the final product that we recognize as.

The amount of CBD oil in the package as milligrams. Sometimes, the label will mention the amount per drop or the dosage per drop.

There's no standardised doses for CBD at the moment. CBD isn't even regulated by the FDA therefore determining precise numbers could be a challenge.

The final decision will depend on several variables, such as:

* The disease being managed

* Your body's weight

• Your health condition level, your lifestyle and exercise intensity

* The level of CBD in every drop of oil

It's best to follow according to a medical recommendation. They'll provide useful advice that is based on your overall health, body chemical composition, as well as the potency of the CBD oil you select to utilize.

If you do not require a prescription from a physician you should start at a low dose, and then increase your dosage gradually. Twenty mg can be a great starting point for mild health problems and up to 40 mg to treat more severe issues like chronic discomfort.

If you don't feel any effect you are not feeling any effect, then increase the dose each week by 5 mg until you feel relief.

Chapter 6: How CBD Oil Affects the Body

CBD oil won't get the same amount of notice if it weren't actually doing something to be noticed!

The majority of CBD positive stories (refer to Chapter 10 for more in-depth tales) resulted in sudden and evident results that were noticed shortly following the first treatment using CBD oil.

There's no doubt about that the power of the compound.

In other forms, cannabis has amazing effects, however CBD oil is the most effective form of CBD to absorb by the body. It will then get working quickly and efficiently.

Human body cells are designed to be responsive to CBD. Like the respiratory system, which is specifically designed to work with air, so too do we have an endocannabinoid system created to work with cannabis.

We haven't ever thought of having such a system in our body. Doesn't this mean that, when used properly, CBD is a perfectly naturally occurring thing to utilize?

The Endocannabinoid System

The endocannabinoid system was an endocannabinoid system that was only discovered inside our body. It was discovered in the 1990s by research scientists who were who were studying THC.

It's crucial to realize that the endocannabinoid process (also called the ECS) is present in each living thing. No matter if you've ever had experiences with marijuana or not, the system is present and serves to fulfill a function.

Scientists can state with relative confidence that the ECS is a factor in:

* Sleep quality

The mood of our hearts are at any moment.

* Our desire to eat

* The power of our memories

* Reduced inflammation

* Regulating metabolism

Effective motor control

While research continues It is generally accepted that the principal role that ECS ECS is to regulate homeostasis throughout the body.

This means that when the external forces alter some thing, the endocannabinoid process is able to bring it back to equilibrium. In the case of experiencing an illness that causes fever, the ECS is working hard to restore your body to the proper temperature.

Components of the Endocannabinoid System

The ECS is comprised of three elements:

* Endocannabinoids

* Receptors for cannabinoid

* Enzymes

Endocannabinoids

Endocannabinoids contain molecules like the cannabinoids that are found in cannabis and hemp. They are produced inside the human body. This is why they're called "endo", meaning "inside."

In contrast to cannabis, which has more than 100 cannabis cannabinoids few endocannabinoids are discovered at the moment.

Anandamide (AEA), and 2-arachidonoylglycerol (2-AG) were the first two, followed by noladin ether, N-arachidonoyl-dopamine, and virodhamine.

The two first ones have been studied by scientists and are aware of the functions they perform inside the human body. Three more have been identified, however there is no consensus about what exactly they are doing.

They are created in the event that the body requires these substances. It is not yet clear the typical levels for every one of the substances.

Anandamide (AEA)

The first endocannabinoid has been discovered and was named by Mechoulam, Devane, and Hanus (n.d.).

2-arachidonoylglycerol (2-AG)

While it was discovered after AEA 2AG was discovered second to AEA. It is the one with the highest concentration that is present at fairly significant amounts within the brain's central nervous system. As with anandamide identified in the laboratory of Raphael Mechoulam, with the aid of his colleague, Shimon Ben-Shabat (National Center for Biotechnology Information 2021).

Cannabinoid Receptors

Receptors can be found all over the body. They bind with them in order to signal that a specific step must be initiated from the ECS.

There are two kinds of receptors:

* CB1 receptors, found within the central nervous system.

* CB2 receptors are located in the peripheral nerve system.

Certain receptors in the body are bound to Endocannabinoids so that they can send an information to the nervous system.

In the case of endocannabinoids, for instance, they might bind with CB1 receptors located in the spine to signify that pain relief is required. In different situations, one may bind with an CB2 cell, signalling that there is inflammation and must be addressed.

It's important to note that THC can bind to receptors better as CBD does! That's one of the main reasons to take CBD along with THC with a small amount when the user isn't looking for the effects of the high.

Enzymes

After the endocannabinoid is done with its work of communicating its message to our nervous system it must be broken into pieces in order to allow the receptor to be open to receiving the latest messages.

It's the job that enzymes perform. The fatty acid-amide hydrolase break down AEA which is attached to receptors. monoacylglycerol acid lipase is responsible for breaking into 2-AG (Raypole and Carter, 2019).

How the Brain Responds to CBD Oil

What we know is that CBD is a drug that targets various receptors within the peripheral and central nervous system.

If a specific receptor is stimulated through the binding of a cannabinoid intracellular signaling pathways get activated, delivering a message to the brain on what is required within the body in order to correct the issue.

How does this play out in particular outcomes?

There are two people who can use droplets in the same bottle to treat two distinct conditions and they can both be beneficial. Why is it that the identical CBD can have different effects?

The receptors it communicates with.

The research is ongoing However, research up to recently have revealed that the impact of CBD depend on the receptor it associates to.

As an example, when the cannabinoid is given to your body with to ease anxiousness, it might attach to a serotonin receptor. This specific pairing signals to the brain that serotonin is required to fight the symptoms of anxiety. This can lead to the reduction of anxiety-related symptoms.

Similar to that, if cannabis is consumed for helping with withdrawal symptoms in situation in addiction connect with opioid receptors and communicate to the brain in order to lessen craving for the drug.

This way we see the fact that CBD does not directly interact in a direct way with brain. The various receptors function as a middleman in relaying the essential signal to the brain for the CBD.

It's also important to understand that CBD doesn't discriminate in regards to diseases or conditions. If you are taking CBD to ease anxiety, and also suffer from an autoimmune condition and both of them will be helped through CBD.

In this way you can observe that the brain just following instructions! If a job description is given, the brain fulfills the requirement. It reacts to the information it's being given and the whole thing is about the interaction between cannabinoids as well as the receptors (Brain Performance Center 2020).

How the Body Responds to CBD Oil

Once we have a better understanding of the connection between cannabinoids and receptors within the body, as well as the ways they communicate messages to brain cells, it is easier to comprehend the next step: how the body responds CBD oil.

In terms of science, as previously mentioned, our body does not respond with CBD or cannabinoids in any way. Instead, it reacts to brain's signals and instructions, which come after the brain has been instructed on what it should do by cannabinoids that are attached to specific receptors.

When the brain receives an alert from a specific receptor for reducing inflammation, it transmits that message to relevant areas within the body i.e. that is, to the immune system. In response, the immune system activates and then does whatever it takes to minimize inflammation.

When the brain is given the signal to create the hormone needed to correct the imbalance in chemistry it is able to do this without questioning. The brain transmits the signal to the area of the body which produces the hormone needed, then the task is completed.

That's why CBD oil can have such broad impacts on our bodies. In the event you drink a drop of CBD the body doesn't understand what you're doing with it. In contrast to traditional medication that has been designed to serve a specific reason, CBD lets cannabinoids loose within the body, allowing them to investigate and determine what requires to be addressed as well as to perform to create magic in the body from there.

If you're using CBD specifically for the purpose of reducing cravings for drugs, like it's likely the pains and aches that you felt in your back have gone away present. Perhaps you've noticed that when you begin your CBD program, you've caught an illness less frequently. You might notice that you're experiencing more energy than you previously to have, without a clear motive.

CBD simply takes a thorough examination of the body's structure, determines what requires aid, and then ensures it connects with the appropriate receptors in order to create the needed modifications.

It is important to recognize that, despite this being the process which CBD employs to generate amazing outcomes, many other variables are also involved. The evidence is clear the fact that CBD does work and evidence of this is abundant.

However, not all brains and bodies are the identical. In certain instances, there could be a gap between the receptors and the brain, leading to messages not being transmitted from one side to the other.

CBD might be amazing for many reasons, but there's always the chance that it won't work as it typically is, due to a myriad of potential issues.

Difference Between CBD Oil and Smoking Cannabis

In the previous article, we have discussed typical methods of extracting CBD from cannabis. You'll notice that there are some methods that are better in comparison to other. Certain extraction techniques leave behind toxic substances, making use of the end product unwise.

CBD oil that's been correctly processed and comes with COA (Certificate of Analysis) is top-quality, fast-acting and typically quite powerful.

However, what is the effect of smoking the flowers in the plant?

Cannabis smoking has been a popular method to take the drug. Prior to CBD oil became popular, smokers were smoking cannabis!

There are some essential things you need to know about smoking cannabis.

"Smoking Cannabis" Generally Refers to the Flower of the Marijuana Plant

The smoke of hemp plants can be a good idea. But, most likely, you won't feel much. There are more efficient and efficient ways to consume CBD Hemp is a great source of CBD, as it contains less THC, which means there won't be this high and head rush.

If you're planning to use cannabis for advantages to your health and not for the euphoria, the difficulty of smoking hemp is that it's basically a that is a trash container. It absorbs almost all the dirt which it's grown in which means that if you're consuming hemp in the way that it is it's likely that you're breathing in lots of harmful substances together with CBD.

Smoking Gets Into Your Bloodstream Quicker

Smoking cigarettes is a highly effective method of introducing cannabinoids to the system swiftly. It is absorbed within minutes after the taking a puff.

Smoking is Less Healthy Than Oils

The main issue associated that comes with marijuana, aside from the risk of inhaling unpleasant substances with hemp is the possibility to have negative consequences.

Smoking an occasional joint won't cause any problem. If you're a frequent smoker and smoking is the preferred method to take in the drug then you're likely to be inhaling carcinogenic and toxic chemicals in the paper as well as the lighter fluid that is involved during the smoking procedure.

Even vaping brings potential health problems. Chemical solvents as well as components of low quality are a serious risk to health.

If a person is burned, the fumes generated can be a source of a range of poisonous chemicals. As a result that smoking cigarettes has, these substances require to be absorbed by the mouth, throat, trachea and into the lungs, which opens the possibility of catching an infection (American Chemical Society 2007b).

CBD oil has very little risk if you purchase it from a reliable manufacturer who extracts CBD from CBD with care. If CBD oil you choose to purchase is certified by a third party, CBD oil you pick has an Certificate of Analysis from a independent third-party tester the product should be safe enough to consume without having to worry about toxins, contamination or any adverse side effects because of substances different from CBD.

CBD Oil Can Give You a High, or Not

The CBD oil you select could contain sufficient THC for you to experience a high. If you're smoking to get buzz, you could gain greater benefits from CBD oil, which also has greater than 0.3 percent THC. It will provide you with an euphoria, as well as the positive health effects of CBD as well as removing the damage that could be caused to your body from smoking.

CBD Oils Gets Into the Bloodstream Fairly Quickly

Although it might not be able to begin to work in just a few seconds similar to smoking, CBD can still be quite effective the majority of oils acting after 20 to 30 minutes of taking it.

What About Edibles?

CBD brownies, gummies, cupcakes, fudge and many other sweets are now a hugely loved method of taking CBD as well as THC.

Edibles have the potential to be extremely effective to help relax effects of CBD and for the high associated with THC.

It takes longer for them to be processed by the body since they are broken down by the liver. The liver is where THC converts to an additional, stronger substance known as 11-hydroxy-THC.

Depends on the person, and how much they've eaten prior to ingestion It could take anywhere between 15 and 2 hours before the effects begin to show up.

There's a small risk that comes from overdosing on food items since the person believes there has any effect. Although there's no risk from overdosing, it could result in a less satisfying sensation and feeling groggy afterwards.

To THC or Not to THC

THC is considered to be the "good stuff." It's the part of cannabis that makes you feel high. provides that high and causes parents to worry about their child becoming addicted to drugs.

There are many ways to obtain CBD either with or without THC. Most CBD oils have trace levels of THC which is lower than 0.3 percentage, which does not provide the same feeling of high.

Some people find that the experience of a high can be a good complement to the benefits for health of CBD. People who smoke marijuana to benefit their health and appreciate the buzz which it brings might be better off using CBD oil and a bit of THC in order to stay away from the negative consequences of smoking marijuana while experiencing a high.

Although THC by itself isn't as safe in the same way as CBD but it has several advantages. It's not all harmful!

Benefits of THC

As a whole, THC has some surprising advantages. In addition to providing a luxurious and euphoric feeling as well, it has these properties:

Pain Relief

THC is a stimulant of serotonin glutamatergic and dopamine receptors. It might be why it can ease pain.

In certain instances in some instances, in some cases, the THC molecules that are bound to receptors triggers a release of analgesic chemical within the brain. Other times there are instances where the THC inhibits the pain signal so that the brain doesn't even know what it is supposed to feel the pain.

It's crucial to realize that THC isn't a cure for what causes the pain. The effect is to ease the pain to allow you to continue your life with no limitations (Russo 2008.).

Eases Nausea

THC is a key ingredient in the treatment of nausea, particularly when it's associated with chemotherapy. THC binds to 5-HT3 receptors in order to reduce the nausea response (Parker and colleagues. in 2011,).

It's a healthy, more secure alternative to synthetic medications to reduce nausea. Many of which can cause negative adverse effects for patients suffering from chemotherapy.

Alleviates Insomnia

The research suggests that taking 15mg THC a half hour prior to getting to sleep can cause an sedative effect (Nicholson and colleagues. (2004)).

An 2008 study suggests that THC may reduce the quantity of REM sleep upon ingestion. This indicates that the majority of sleep time is during the sleep phase that promotes more relaxation and healing (Schierenbeck and co. (2008)).

There is no need to take an enormous amount of THC in order to make it efficient in helping with insomnia. If you smoke only a couple of puffs of smoke can help.

The THC content also depends to some extent on the type that marijuana is derived from. THC was obtained. In general, THC comes from one of three types: indica, which is relaxing, sativa which stimulates the senses, or hybrids, which could be any of the three.

Improves Appetite

THC can be an effective treatment for eating disorders in addition to patients suffering from ailments that cause them to don't take their food (such with dementia) or lose appetite (such as HIV).

If you've tried marijuana, you're aware of the fact the feeling of "the munchies" is a frequent side consequence. For those who are who are healthy the use of marijuana regularly can cause weight gain, and even weight gain, since the THC is a receptor agonist that can stimulate the appetite.

People who want to keep an increase in appetite can benefit significantly from this technique, and start to get appetite without feeling made to take in food (Hull 2019).

Antioxidant Properties

As with its cousin CBD, THC demonstrates high anti-inflammatory and antioxidant properties.

The process of oxidative stress takes place in our bodies when the ratio of antioxidants and free radicals gets tilted. Free radicals are able to interact with other molecules within the body. This could cause sudden and explosive chemical chain reactions that occur in the body.

The reactions can be beneficial, however they could also cause harm. Antioxidants stabilize free radicals and hinders chain reactions that are sudden from happening.

THC provides antioxidants that can neutralize free radicals and stop large-scale chemical reactions throughout the body. It can lower blood pressure, regulate blood sugar levels as well as reduce inflammation.

Muscle Relaxation

Patients suffering from neuropathic or musculoskeletal muscular pain may be benefited by THC's calming properties.

The research has shown that marijuana eases muscle spasticity by loosing them in order to prevent cramps and shaking.

It's believed to be beneficial for people suffering from Parkinson's disease and multiple sclerosis because of this (Mack and Joy 2000).

THC and Anxiety

THC to treat anxiety is a hot topic. Since THC provides users with an elevated feeling, the effects depend mostly on the user's state of mind before and throughout the use.

If a person is susceptible to anxiety, taking overuse of THC may cause anxiety, and possibly fear and paranoia.

If the person is happy and relaxed prior to beginning to take THC the drug, it's more likely to intensify those feelings after getting the user is high.

Research supports the idea that a low level of THC could improve the signs of anxiety. There's a lot of evidence to suggest that THC may increase anxiety (Parmet 2017.).

It usually depends on the dosage as well as the individual's body's chemical. Most likely, a mixture of CBD as well as THC will be the most effective way for relieving anxiety, as well as low-dose THC will more likely work than higher doses.

The Case for THC

The advantages of THC can be seen. However, there's a thin boundary between when the use of high dosages is more beneficial or detrimental.

Whatever the case, evidence for the effect of the entourage indicates that CBD is more potent in combination with THC in smaller doses (HealthMed 2020).

People looking to experience a buzz will find one that has the additional benefits that come with CBD. If you want to reap the advantages of the effects on the body however, but not experience the high may still enjoy it by using the low dose THC products. These are those in which the THC concentration is below 0.3 percentage.

It's only fitting to delve into the impact of CBD on cancer in the beginning since my personal story has been one of beating disease through CBD oil.

The cancer statistics are scary. Cancer is the second most common causes of death in the world and accounts for 1 out of 6 deaths worldwide (World Health Organization, 2018,).

It's not just a single disease also. There are a variety of illnesses that cause problems to any part of the body. They can also display various indicators and signs.

Cancer is especially dangerous because we do not have the full picture of the causes and cures for it. Certain aspects are determining if someone is a good potential candidate to get cancer, however, it is possible to affect people that are healthy like it is able to be avoided by those who appear to be a good candidate.

The term "cancer" refers to the normal, healthy cells within the body transform into cancer cells. This can be a long-term process.

The chances of developing cancer depend on genes and

* Carcinogens that are physical (cancer-causing pathogens) such as ultraviolet light

* Biological carcinogens such as bacteria or viruses

* Carcinogens from chemicals, such as nicotine smoke toxins

Although a balanced lifestyle may help prevent cancer to a degree but an "perfect storm" of genetics and carcinogen exposure could cause cancer cells to develop anywhere at any point.

The most commonly encountered kinds of cancer include cancers of the breast, lung, colorectal and prostate cancer, as well as skin as well as stomach cancer. Of course, every type is extremely dangerous and may cause death, however we'll focus on CBD to help you recognize the most popular varieties.

If you have a form of cancer that's not mentioned in this guide CBD oil might provide a viable treatment. Consult your physician first. If they're not convinced (which there are still some) seeking a second opinion or locating a CBD specialist near you is ideal.

Brain Cancer

I've witnessed the positive benefits of CBD for brain cancer in my own personal experience. In addition to my experience of my personal experience it is clear that there's plenty of research on the impact CBD is having on brain cancer particularly glioblastoma one of the most dangerous type of cancer that available (American Brain Tumor Association, 2018.).

There are no good statistics for the glioblastoma. About five percent of those who are diagnosed with the disease survive for more than five years. Nearly 75% die within a year after having been diagnosed.

Recent studies have shown remarkable results using pharmaceutical grade CBD or CBD/THC for treating cancerous glioblastomas. The untreated group, which didn't receive CBD, had a survival rate of 44% within one year. The CBD group that received THC was amazed by the increase in survival rate by the time they reached the 1 year date, which was 83 percent (Dumitru and co. 2018, 2018).

Another research study yielded intriguing findings. From 119 patients only 28 patients received CBD as their sole therapy and others were given CBD in addition to their previous treatment. CBD was administered in a three-day on 3 days off and for at least six months. The dosage vary based on the extent of cancer.

Some patients, however, went to using CBD oil that they purchased from the internet, and, in those instances the majority were relapsed. An example of this was one patient aged five who's anaplastic brain tumor diminished to 60 percent within 10 months.

A patient aged 50 with advanced tanycytic ependymoma grade 2 displayed an improvement in the tumor size within 6 months of using the synthetic pharmaceutical grade CBD in the aftermath of making the change from traditional oncology medications. When the test was conducted the patient began making use of the CBD extract purchased online and after a year the tumor had increased in dimensions (Kenyon and co. 2018, 2018).

How CBD Works on Brain Cancer

Studies are underway on the CBD isolate that is 100% CBD isolate as well as CBD extract (with tiny levels of THC). Both produced similar results, in such a way that researchers consider the difference to be not significant.

Researchers believe that CBD interacts with receptors in order to focus on mitochondria, vital to our body cells. Injecting CBD to mitochondria seems to cause them to fail in the end, which eventually leads to their death in a way that causes the cell to die (Experimental Biology 2020). You can imagine CBD can prove extremely beneficial in the reduction of cancerous cells.

The latest research suggests CBD may have a positive impact on itself, however, it can also improve the effect of chemotherapy. Patients who aren't willing to go through chemotherapy could be able to benefit from medical-grade CBD and has an added benefit of none of the adverse consequences.

It's crucial to know that CBD supplements that you can purchase online appear to be ineffective or had no impact on the brain cancer cells in these studies. The pharmaceutical-grade CBD products could be the only method for CBD to prove effective against cancer of the brain.

Breast Cancer

Breast cancer is among the most prevalent kinds of cancer. It is a possibility for women and men however it is more common for women. The cancer forms tumors and may be spread to other organs when not addressed early enough.

CBD has demonstrated evidence of it being beneficial for a number different purposes in treating breast cancer. But CBD is certainly more effective prior to cancer has metastrate.

A study from 2019 has revealed that CBD may help reduce cancer size, and also slows the development of breast cancer cells as well as helps to prevent metastasis (McAllister and colleagues. in 2011,).

Even though CBD has been proven to reduce tumors and stopping the cancer from spreading and spreading to other areas, there is evidence that a lot of breast cancer patients take CBD for managing adverse effects and signs they experience due to treatments or radiation (Nurgali and colleagues. in 2018,).

Research has shown that some patients have been successful using CBD to treat nausea and vomiting in addition to pain, anorexia, loss of appetite as well as anxiety and stress that are associated with the condition (Weiss and colleagues. (2020).

How CBD Works on Breast Cancer

There's a myriad of ways CBD is beneficial for patients with breast cancer. When it comes to treating cancer, it seems that it isn't often utilized in isolation, rather as an adjunct treatment alongside conventional radiation and chemotherapy.

The anti-tumor properties of CBD are among reasons CBD is especially effective in treating cancers like breast cancer, where tumors form major components of the illness. Similar to brain cancer, CBD reduces the mass of tumors in breast cancer because it targets cancer mitochondria in the cancer cells, causing the cells to die.

Along with also reducing the size of tumors, CBD shows significant promise for preventing metastasis or the spread of cancer across different organs. Research has revealed over the years the genes which is the reason for sharing cancerous cells across organs and this gene is called the gene Id-1.

The primary role of this gene lies in cell differentiation. It is that it transforms one kind of cell into another kind. When breast cancer patients are diagnosed Id-1 causes healthy cells that are normal to change into cancerous ones within the breast tissues.

CBD is shown to be an inhibitor of Id-1. CBD blocks the typical speedy growth of cancer cells, which causes metastasis (McAllister and co. 2011, 2011b Caffarel et. al. (2012)).

Cancer patients with breast cancer receiving chemotherapy or radiation treatment will likely suffer certain negative side results of this treatment which include nausea, loss appetite and in more severe instances, tissue and nerve injury that causes neuropathic pain.

As we've previously discussed, CBD molecules function by binding to receptors inside the body, and transmitting signals to the brain regarding what to do about signs. The way in which CBD works CBD in dealing with these symptoms is dependent on the symptoms, since various receptors are responsible for a variety of issues.

However, using the pharmaceutical grade CBD has proven to be effective in for reducing nausea and gastric disturbances as a consequence of chemo therapy, increasing appetite and offering relief from chronic pain that results from nerve injury or tissue.

Prostate Cancer

Prostate cancer is among the most frequent cancer among American males and is also among the most significant cancers that cause death worldwide.

Unexpectedly, prostate cancer cells are replete with cannabinoid receptors. So CBD could be a powerful tool when it comes to this form of cancer, too.

There are more research studies on prostate cancer as well as CBD over other kinds of cancer, the initial study shows that CBD is a similar effect on prostate cancers just as it does with other tumors (Singh and co. in 2020).

There's evidence to suggest that CBD blocks the exomes released by prostate cancer cell (Sperling 2020). Exomes contain molecules that send messages from and to cells, and they can alter their behaviour in response to these signals. They can also hinder the development of cells.

Additionally, CBD containing THC helps to stop the development of vital blood vessels within cancer, which prevents the tumor from getting nourished and expanding.

At present, there aren't any human clinical trials on this. The only clinical studies in connection with prostate cancer as well as CBD are ones that focus on managing symptoms of pain as well as the adverse consequences of chemotherapy, in which CBD has proven to be a strong proof that it is a successful treatment to treat adverse negative effects.

How CBD Works on Prostate Cancer

Prostate cancer cells react well to cannabinoids. They are able to respond well CB1 as well as CB2 receptors found in prostate cancer are extremely receptive to cannabinoids. They will also connect with them in other cancerous cells.

This enables CBD to target cancer cells. CBD to attack cancer cells, which when given cannabinoids treatment, are more likely to self-destruct.

Research suggests that CBD decreases the activities of the androgen receptors found in cancer cells. Androgens are hormones that aid male traits While they're essential to ensure the health of the prostate gland, they are also vital in the development and growth of cancerous prostate cells (National Cancer Institute, 2019.).

Prostate cancer typically is managed with a drug that stops the production of testosterone, or surgically removing the testicles (which takes out the orrogen-producing cells completely) or by removing the testicular tissue which produce androgens.

CBD treatment has proven to be capable of decreasing androgen receptor activities within cancerous cells. This signifies that the cancer cells have been removed from the right environment to live and grow. Cancer cells start to fade away.

In addition to being helpful in reducing tumors and inhibiting androgens CBD is also a great aid to patients with prostate cancer to ease the pain that comes with treating their disease. The side effects of treatment, like damaged nerves or muscle within the prostate region or neuropathic pain nausea that is associated with treatment may be alleviated with the help CBD oil. CBD oil.

Another common side effect from prostate cancer include the erectile dysfunction as well as urinary incontinence. Though they are likely due to muscle or damaged tissue, CBD could be a beneficial treatment.

The efficacy of CBD in treating these diseases depends in large part on the underlying cause. Certain research studies point to the possibility the Ayurvedic practitioners have utilized cannabis for thousands of years to boost sexual health, however scientists of today aren't certain the way it could assist.

There's an idea that it can relax blood vessels to improve penis circulation however, to date it's not clear and quick information about the way it could differ in the case of prostate cancer, and when its typical treatments are being used (Chauhan and colleagues. (2014)).

Lung Cancer

Lung cancer is among the most prevalent cancers which is why 15 percent of those suffering from lung cancer aren't smokers.

There are two kinds of lung cancers: non-small-cell lung cancer that makes up 80% of lung cancers. There is also small-cell bronchial cancer, which makes about 20% of all instances.

Small-cell cancer is the most aggressive kind, and tumors can develop fast. It also metastasises quickly. The non-small-cell types of tumors consist of bigger cells and tend to be only present in one part of the lung. They also tend to shrink slower.

Non-small-cell tumors are surgically eliminated with minimal adverse negative effects. Chemotherapy should only be considered if another organ has been damaged.

Small-cell tumors can spread to other areas in around 70% of the cases. This makes them challenging to cure. Most often, chemotherapy or radiotherapy are the only treatments available.

The study of CBD for a possible alternative treatment for cancer of the lung is in its early days. The clinical trials are currently being planned. If we look at CBD's function when it comes to other cancers We can conclude that CBD works in similar to the way it affects the growth of lung cancer tumors.

A case study on an 81 year old lung cancer patient who had an area of 2,5 cm x 2,5 cm tumor demonstrated significant improvement through treatment using CBD oil.

The patient refused treatment with radiotherapy and chemotherapy however, he decided to treat himself by using an online-purchased 200mg CBD oil. It started by taking two drops a day, and then increased to 9 drops per day within a week.

Then, he stopped his treatment for over a month then self-treated using 9 drops of CBD oil per every day for over the course of a month before taking a break from the CBD oil treatment completely. An examination three months later found the tumor approximately 10% its size (Sule-Suso and colleagues. in 2019,).

It is important to remember that the patient did not make any modifications to their lifestyles or diets or underwent any other therapies. It's a hopeful study to determine the future of cancer treatments for lung cancer using CBD!

How CBD Works on Lung Cancer

As lung cancer is a type of cancer that causes tumors, its effect by CBD in treating the disease is comparable to the effects on other cancers that cause tumors. CBD is believed to reduce tumors because of its anti-cancer qualities.

The research suggests that CBD can be used on a variety of ways to diminish cancerous cells. In particular, CBD appears to enhance the likelihood of the process of apoptosis (cell death) within cancer cells (ChoiPark and co. in 2008).

Additionally, (and various other functions within our bodies), CBD inhibits the creation and function of tumor-related macrophages. It also enhances the vulnerability of cancer cells destroyed by the immune system.

Leukemia

Leukemia is among the cancers with the greatest variety and has a variety of kinds. It's a condition that affects the blood-forming tissue, which can cause damage to blood cells and the bone marrow. There are four major forms of leukemia. However, there are many mutations.

Unlike most cancers, leukemia doesn't form tumors. Regarding shrinking tumor size or inhibiting expansion of tumor cells CBD isn't able to treat leukemia in the same manner it affects other kinds of cancer.

Leukemia usually affects the white blood cells. These form an essential component in the immune system. They combat foreign objects. When a person is affected by leukemia, white blood cells perform differently and fail to do the job they are supposed to do. The abnormal cells be extremely prolific, ultimately blocking healthy blood cells.

Studies have shown that CBD can be a potent and efficient treatment for leukemia. There are research suggesting that maximum potency could be attained in combination therapy along with chemotherapy (Scott and colleagues. 2017.).

One striking illustration that shows the power of CBD as a whole is in a study from 2013 that shows the development of a patient aged 14 who was suffering from acute lymphoblastic Leukemia (ALL) that was made more aggressive due to the Philadelphia Chromosome mutation.

The patient received an organ transplantation as well as chemotherapy and radiation therapy. All that were found to be unfavorable. After the treatment lasted for 34 months, the patient was transferred into palliative care, and was deemed as terminal after following the exhaustion of conventional therapies.

In just two weeks, the patient has received a prescription that included hemp oil. Hemp oil differs from the traditional CBD oil, in that it is made from the seeds rather than the substance in the plant. The cannabinoid remains.

It was suspended with honey an antibacterial and natural digestive soother. It was administered with increasing dosages every day for 15 consecutive days. On Day 6, number of blast cells in the patient's body began to decline. The following day the second hemp oil type was added. After an initial surge in blast cell counts the numbers decreased steadily to nearly the level of 0.

The infection in the central line was identified on the day 41. This led to hospitalization as well as a dosage of antibiotics. The days 44-49, with hemp oil strain number three, did not show any increase blast cell count.

Between the days of 50 and 67, there was the growth of blast cell number, a phenomenon that coincided with the patient getting sick from refeeding syndrome as well as the body being in shock as a result of being treated by antibiotics. From days 69 to 788, the blast cells of the patient decrease to nearly 0.

While the patient died due to the effects of the compromised immune system it is evident that the use of cannabinoids showed a remarkable result on an allegedly terminal illness (Singh and Bali 2013).

How CBD Works on Leukemia

Although leukemia isn't associated with cancerous tumors, CBD still works on killing cancerous cells. The research conducted as long to 2005 has shown that CBD caused cell death and apoptosis in leukemia cells (Powles and co. 2005).

CBD works with CB receptors that in turn trigger cell Apoptosis within the unusual white blood cells (McKallip 2006). Evidence suggests CBD and THC interact to CBD as well as THC inhibit the development of cancer cells so they do not reach maturity (Murison and colleagues. 1987).

They are effective in their own right, however research suggests the most effective method consisting of CBD addition and chemotherapy maybe because CBD reduces side effect of chemotherapy as well as helps to speed up healing.

Naturally, like other types of cancer, CBD is effective at combating chemo-related side effects when patients are undergoing standard treatment.

While colorectal cancer is among the third-most frequent cancer, there's not much evidence that suggests CBD helping to reduce it.

Colon as well as rectal cancer can be two distinct illnesses. However, one of them can lead to another, and they're often described in conjunction as colorectal tumors.

However, research has produced interesting results for the other 10 cannabinoids, in addition to CBD and THC when it comes to lab tests with synthetic cannabinoids. They appeared to stop the growth of cancer cells, however, CBD as well as THC were not able to affect the growth of cancer cells (Penn State, 2019,).

However, other studies show that CBD can indeed decrease the size of tumors and impedes the proliferation of cancerous cells that cause colorectal cancer (Aviello and al. (2012); Romano et al. 2014).

How CBD Works on Colorectal Cancer

As with other types of cancer the colorectal cancer manifests with the development of abnormally-shaped tumors and cells.

CBD and THC trigger THC and CBD stimulate CB1 as well as CB2 receptors. These trigger specific actions within the body. These actions target cancerous cells, and making them disintegrate from the inside.

Regular usage of CBD may also help alleviate conditions that occur as the result of traditional treatment, like treatment with radiation or chemotherapy. CBD can help boost the immune system while keeping the inflammation at bay, which can result in less difficulty in the face of illness (Croxford and Yamamura in 2005).

Stomach Cancer

Stomach cancer may develop within the primary area of the stomach. However, in the USA the majority of them develop at the point in the stomach where it meets the esophagus.

The site of the cancer could determine the outcome for treatment. Sometimes surgeries can be beneficial. For others treatment, radiation or chemotherapy may be the best option.

Stomach cancer is a result of the cell becoming different, and the cell does not behave as the normal stomach cells. The affected cell becomes more massive than normal. It is also able to survive in the event that normal cells die.

It's not long before new cells to transform in the process, and when they grow in a tumour, they develop that may be able to recruit healthy cells or eliminate them. Stomach cancer may also spread into other organs.

The results of studies on mice show the fact that CBD is not only a deterrent to the proliferation of cancer cells but also helps reduce the dimensions of cancerous tumors. Researchers used a synthetic cannabis that was administered to mice, and those who were treated with it saw one-third reduction to 30 percent in the size of their tumors within just 15 days (Jeong and colleagues. 2019, 2019).

The studies on human gastric cancer tissue cells have shown an important reduction in cell proliferation and rise in cell apoptosis after being treatment with CBD (Zhang and co. in 2019,).

Research suggests that CBD could be an effective treatment for stomach cancer while also decreasing gastric discomfort as well as the side consequences of treatments.

How CBD Works on Stomach Cancer

In general, the manner in which cancers grow is similar regardless of the region in which body they form. They develop abnormally, grow in a way that is unusually fast, and eventually form groups that is what makes them a cancer. This then starts to impact the surrounding cells by making them tumor-like cells or infusing them with.

CBD is a normal function to treat these cells that are abnormal. Through binding to CB1 or CB2 receptors the growth of abnormal cells is diminished, and finally cell Apoptosis occurs, which causes cancer cells to go out of existence and allow healthier ones to replace them.

It also assists in preventing the spread of cancerous tumors different organs, making cancer less difficult to treat.

Stomach cancer is a cause of various gastric symptoms including an increase in appetite and weight loss, nausea nausea, abdominal pain, nausea, as well as indigestion. each of which has been found to be efficiently treated with CBD.

Skin Cancer

Skin cancer is present in many different methods. Most often, it occurs on areas exposed to sun light however, it may occur anywhere on the body too.

It could appear as an oblique bump of wax at the top of the skin, or as a sloping or growing mole skin lesion that it forms a crust it could be a smaller cut that isn't healing.

They are caused by an cells that are not growing normally in the skin's top layer. skin. The cause can be caused by UV radiation or exposure to toxins or conditions of the immune system.

In certain instances, people who've received radiotherapy for cancers of other types are more at risk of being diagnosed with skin cancer as a result of being exposed to radiation.

CBD oil could be an effective cure for the disease and signs and symptoms that accompany it. The skin, which is the biggest organ inside the body has CB receptors as well. If you apply CBD cream or oil to the surface, they absorb it to the skin without being required to be absorbed into the bloodstream initially.

There is plenty of evidence to support CBD helping with inflammatory disorders, which includes irritation of the skin (Scheau and colleagues. 2010).

There are other studies that show CBD as well as other cannabinoids preventing the proliferation of cancerous cells, decreasing circulation of blood to tumors and stopping the growth of tumor cells (Casanova and co. 2003).

How CBD Works on Skin Cancer

CBD is available in a variety of ways to treat skin cancer. First, it is cosmetic creams and other products that are applied to the skin on the spot of cancer. CBD oil is effective also in this manner. They are absorbed straight from the point of origin and do not need to be absorbed into the bloodstream before they can be absorbed.

Tinctures, edibles and oils are able to be consumed by mouth, either in the form of drops or as active ingredients in meals. The mucous membranes of the mouth take them in rapidly and it doesn't take for long to begin becoming effective.

It's crucial to keep in mind that even though applying CBD directly on the skin could seem like the ideal method of treatment however, there are other methods that could be equally efficient. Each works in the exact identical way. They all interact with receptors in order to trigger specific body reactions.

CBD oil that is taken orally may also help with the pain that results from the illness, as well as additional side effects may appear. CBD creams are not as efficient for treatment or treatment of any negative side consequences.

Conclusion

There's no doubt about the fact that CBD whether on it's own or with other traditional cancer therapies, will effectively shrink the size and volume of tumors as well with other cancerous cells throughout the body.

Though all cancers are somewhat different, CBD works the same method for all cancers--targeting cells that divide and change improperly, causing Apoptosis as well as stopping the growth of and spreading.

It's worthwhile adding an amount of CBD in cancer treatment regardless of whether it's due to its capacity to ease nausea and vomiting. Additionally, it can reduce anxiety.

Chapter 7: CBD for Neurological Disorders

It's not the only issue for which CBD can do wonders for. There is still a lot of research to be done as to the effect of CBD treatment on a wide range of neurologic disorders, and certain studies showing remarkably positive outcomes.

Neurological disorders are conditions that impact the brain or nerves. They could be a result of structural causes caused by the structure of the brain, or result from electrical or biochemical abnormalities within the brain.

The causes are numerous and diverse They can appear from nowhere and impact people who seem to be well. Researchers are still discovering a lot about many of these ailments.

It's crucial to understand the distinction between disorders of the neurological and psychiatric. These disorders manifest as a physical manifestation that affects the brain and body and psychiatric or mental disorders are conditions where feeling and thinking, as well as behavior are impaired. It can cause stress in the patients and, in rare situations, a decline in the person's ability to function normally.

A few neurological diseases result from genetic influences. Genetic disorders are present during the pregnancy before birth. Some may result from various other causes, like injuries, exposure to toxins and even cancer.

Traditional medical professionals must be very cautious regarding treating neurological diseases because the root of the problem must be addressed prior to the signs appear, CBD offers a secure alternative that treats many aspects within the neurological condition with little or none negative adverse side adverse effects (WHO Team 2016).

There isn't a comprehensive coverage of all disorders of the brain in this guide. It is however safe to presumed that CBD will have a beneficial impact on almost any neurological disease you could imagine.

It's a good idea to consult with your physician before contemplating the addition of CBD to your treatment regimen (Russo 2018, 2018).

Epilepsy

Epilepsy's reaction to CBD oil is the topic of a lot of research in these past years. Epilepsy is a neurologic disorder where the patient suffers frequent and sometimes severe seizures.

It's among the five most frequent neurological diseases, and isn't discriminatory. It affects people of any age and gender. One may be predisposed to the condition if they've got an inheritance pattern in their family, or they have an increased risk of developing the condition after brain trauma or exposure to toxic substances. In the majority of cases, but the root of epilepsy remains a mystery.

Seizures are caused due to abnormal electrical activity within the brain. There are two kinds of seizures. They are generalized that affects the whole brain as well as focal which just affect a specific part of the brain.

In between the two, there are various types of seizures. Some that cause lack of consciousness, and others that are not noticeable.

There are many ways epilepsy can be addressed. It is largely dependent upon the extent of the condition and the way of life of the individual affected.

* Anticonvulsant drugs

This is the most popular treatment for epilepsy. In certain cases it is possible to eliminate seizures entirely, but most of the time they drastically reduce the frequency of seizures a patient experiences every day, as well as restore some regularity to their lives.

Like all chemical medications using these, it is possible to result in unwanted reactions. Though seizures could become a thing of in the past, some users begin suffering from sleepiness nausea, dizziness, weight loss or increase and fatigue, as well as irritability as well as anxiety and depression, trouble concentrating, gastric disturbance, blurred vision or balance issues among others.

Alternative treatment options include:

* Brain surgery

In the event of severe seizures If they are severe, the area of the brain affected may be taken out. However, who would like to eliminate a portion or their entire brain? The procedure could have negative side effects, such as a change in character or memory loss, or even confusion.

* Vagus nerve stimulator

The implanted device, which is surgically placed in the chest is able to stimulate the autonomic nerve which runs through the neck before reaching the brain. This may help decrease or prevent seizures. This is an in-depth procedure but it could result in other issues.

* Ketogenic diet

There is evidence that suggests those suffering from epilepsy could benefit from ketogenic diets. This isn't a cure for epilepsy, however, it may help in reducing seizures due to a rise in fat acids (Pietrangelo 2014.).

CBD as an Alternative Treatment

Contrary to conventional remedies, CBD presents a safer alternative to medication that doesn't suffer from negative side effects that can be fatal.

The effects of CBD on the drug-resistant types of epilepsy including Dravet Syndrome and Lennox Gastaut syndrome are well-documented (Severe myoclonic Epilepsy of Childhood--An overview n.d. Lennox-Gastaut syndrome--An Overview, n.d.).

The instances of Charlotte Figi and Alfie Dingley are receiving a lot of attention and show clearly the potential of CBD in restoring normality to the lives of patients in severe and crippling epilepsy.

A study conducted in 2016 of over 100 epilepsy patients between one and 30 found proof that CBD can reduce seizures by more than 40 percent (Devinsky and co. 2016,).

Similar to other disorders the use of CBD from pharmaceutical grade is proven far more effective than CBD for reducing seizures.

It's important to note that the treatment known as Epidiolex(r) was accepted by FDA. It is a CBD-rich product that has 100mg per milliliter. Its main components are flavoring oils, sesame seeds, as well as dehydrated alcohol. This is an encouraging indicator of the potential for CBD as a feasible treatment choice.

Alzheimer's Disease

Alzheimer's disease is a neurologic disease that can affect the brain and memory. It's crucial to recognize what the difference is between Alzheimer's and dementia. It's not a condition by itself, it's an illness type. It's the general term for conditions that impact the mental condition. Alzheimer's disease is a form of dementia.

The disease is slow-growing and the majority of people show mild signs as they reach their late 60s. It's actually called late-onset Alzheimer's and early-onset patients showing indications from 30 and up.

Initial symptoms are insignificant. The time frame can be as long as 10 years before classic cognitive and memory issues show up. Initial signs are slight memory loss, which can lead to a loss of things or getting lost in their normal route, bad judgment and difficulties making choices, mood or personality changes as well as an increase in aggression or anxiety.

As the illness progresses, memory loss becomes more severe regular activities like writing, reading and conversing, become increasingly challenging. Inattention problems and difficulty in organizing and explaining their thinking process may follow.

The paranoia can set in and hallucinations are not unusual. The sufferer may not be able to identify their family or friends or engage in bizarre or inappropriate behaviors like removing their clothes in public, or uttering outbursts of inappropriate speech.

In the advanced stage of the disease, brain tissue is shrinking noticeably and the body starts to slow down because it becomes unable to complete tasks it's required to (National Institute of Aging, 2019.).

How Can CBD Oil Help?

At present, there's no method to reverse the harm caused by Alzheimer's. As it takes 10 years for Alzheimer's to manifest itself the disease, it is difficult to recognize in the early stages. Also, there is no way to stop the spread of the illness in its tracks. However, the research on it has increased over the last few years.

CBD is definitely not an effective treatment for Alzheimer's or other forms of dementia. CBD is commonly employed to treat the neuropsychiatric signs of the condition, which includes depression, anxiety as well as aggression, sleep and eating disorders and obsessional compulsive behaviour.

The use of conventional medications can aggravate signs or trigger additional side consequences. In this light, CBD as an alternative to conventional medicine is currently being thought of.

In contrast to other diseases we've discussed it doesn't show the growth of cells. It causes neurons in the brain to deteriorate, which causes the brain to lose memories as well as learned behavior.

In this instance rather than relying on cell apoptosis characteristics, CBD employs its neuroprotective capabilities. Research has shown that CBD can protect cells against damage to the neuron and also oxidative stress (Kim and co. 2019, 2019) and also promotes neurogenesis, also known as new cell expansion within the brain (Esposito and others. 2011,).

Research suggests that a mix of CBD as well as THC might be a great option solution for neurological disorders. It's crucial to keep in mind however, that CBD can be used to enhance your quality of life of Alzheimer's patients, but is not an effective treatment.

Neuropathic Pain

The pain of neuropathic can be hard to comprehend, since it is very real, but frequently is not accompanied by a specific reason. The somatosensory system is at risk composed of neuronal pathways as well as sensory neurons which respond to the external and internal stimulus external, and trigger certain responses inside the body.

Imagine that you kick your toe over the leg of your table. The nerves that run through your toe communicate all the way to your brain telling it to inform it that something happened and requires a pain-reaction. The brain will then relay the message down to the nerves that they feel discomfort. The whole process takes only a few seconds, however it occurs as a consequence of an moment; in this instance you have smashed your toe.

When you experience neuropathic pain there's no cause. The nerves just emit pain signals with no reason. The result is the sensation of pain, which does not have a reason. It is therefore very difficult to manage.

There are three factors that could create neuropathic pain

* Disease

* Injury

* Infection

Conditions like diabetes, cancer as well as nerve disorders are known to cause chronic pain. Tumors that are cancerous may not be visible however they press against nerves and cause pain for apparent no cause. It can also damage nerves and cause pain to various regions of the body and most often, it is the feet and legs.

Chemotherapy, alcohol abuse radiation, and chemotherapy can affect nerves. This could result in chronic neuropathic discomfort.

Injuries and accidents can cause nerve damage. In some cases, nerves are damaged as a result of the accident which can lead to a long-lasting, chronic painful. In some cases the scar tissue grew and put pressure on nerves, which is not seen, yet very strongly experienced.

Chronic pain from an infection is not common. There are some certain infections that may cause this, which include syphilis, shingles, as well as HIV (Holland and Moawad the year 2020).

The final condition that could cause persistent neuropathic pain is referred to as Phantom leg syndrome. This happens after a limb is amputated. The nerves that are near the site of amputation may malfunction because of trauma and emit signals which the brain interpret as originating from the lost leg. The sufferers experience pain when there's no part of their body!

CBD as a Treatment for Chronic Neuropathic Pain

It's unclear the reason or method by which CBD can help alleviate neuropathy pain. The reasons for chronic pain may not be obvious, it's difficult to determine what issues need to be taken care of.

There's evidence to suggest to suggest that CBD is a glycine receptor antagonist as well as, through its interactions results in an analgesic or sedative effect (Xiong and co. (2012)).

A second study has provided solid proof of the efficacy of THC/CBD as supplement to spinal stimulation in patients who suffer from neuropathy pain due to unsuccessful back surgery.

Eleven patients avoided conventional treatments, with the exception of spinal cord stimulation. Then, they began taking supplements with CBD as a treatment complement.

The majority of the patients reported successful relief from pain for a time of 12 months, using only CBD as a pain reliever. One of the most notable results was the pain perception of patients that was measured using an instrument before the study began that was lowered from an initial value of 8.18 + 1.07 up to 4.72 + 0.9 when the study had come to a close (Mondello and co. 2018,).

CBD oil that is taken orally in drinks or mixed with food can prove effective in treating all forms of neuropathy. A study on animals showed some evidence suggesting that CBD cream or oil applied on the skin may be an analgesic, as well (Grinspoon (2018)).

Parkinson's Disease

Parkinson's is a degenerative disease that impacts the nervous system and how the body moves. The main signs of Parkinson's disease are:

* Tenseness (especially on the limbs, jaw, and the head)

Stiffness of the limbs and body and limbs, which can be accompanied by a loss of facial expression.

• Impaired balance and coordination

The slowing down of normal movement patterns, such as those that are commonplace

Other indications that could occur due to stiff muscles include difficulties swallowing and chewing, slurred speech, a shift in pitch or vocal tone, difficulty in defecating and urinating, sleeping problems, anxiety, and depression.

Body functions that usually are autonomous might start to cause problems. The heart rate and blood pressure vary, and chronic fatigue as well as neuropathy are typical along with a decrease in smell is frequently observed.

Parkinson's disease is the result of the cells that produce dopamine in the brain that die in a manner that is unusually rapid. Dopamine is among the happy chemicals found in the brain and functions as a messenger for the molecular system to other parts of the body. One of the contributing factors could have to do with a lack of norepinephrine. This hormone controls dopamine.

Dopamine levels are reduced and levels drop, your body to respond in a variety of unusual and strange methods that are not under the body's control. who is living within the body.

People suffering from Parkinson's are treated by the use of medications as well as lifestyle modifications. Resting enough, eating an appropriate diet and working out whenever it is it is possible are key elements of the therapy regimen.

The medical field falls into one of the following categories:

* Levodopa, a dopamine replenisher

* Dopamine-based agonists, that are similar to dopamine's effects

* Anticholinergics inhibit the autonomic nervous system.

* COMT inhibitors. It are used to delay the effects of Levodopa.

MAO B inhibitors which degrade the dopamine that is found in the brain.

Each one of them comes with its own set of side negative effects. Like, Levodopa, the most commonly used Parkinson's medication, could result in the development of low blood pressure as well as nausea and vomiting. Due to this, it is often prescribed with a different medication known as carbidopa and makes use of chemicals in addition to the other chemicals.

Certain COMT inhibitors could result in liver damage. MAO B inhibitors are known to cause adverse interactions with other drugs. Also, it is recommended not to discontinue the use of Levodopa abruptly or without the direction of your physician because it could cause serious medical problems.

If medication isn't working The next option is to stimulate the brain deep. It involves surgically affixing electrodes on the brain, and attaching them to the electronic device that is embedded into the chest. As a pacemaker, this device is able to stimulate your cerebrum (painlessly) and reduces the tremors. This is an insidious and last-resort treatment.